Blessings in the Womb

A Prayer Handbook for Pregnant Women

With Post-Partum Recovery Prayers

By
Olu Wonders

DEDICATION

This prayer book is dedicated to all women who are blessed with the fruit of the womb, who passed through the beautiful nine months of pregnancy carrying another human being in their body. You are doing well, and you have done a great job.

CONTENTS

INTRODUCTION

Welcome to "Blessings in the Womb: A Prayer Handbook for Pregnant Women." This book is designed to be a companion and guide for expectant mothers, offering a collection of heartfelt prayers and verses to nurture the spiritual journey of pregnancy.

Having experienced the tasking and beautiful journey of pregnancy and delivery, I recognize the importance of prayers for pregnant women during and after pregnancy, it takes the grace of God to get pregnant and deliver successfully. From the moment when conception is established, the fetus is already a human being in the sight of God. Mothers must carefully invest in the destiny of their children even before they are born.

Pregnancy is a remarkable season of life, filled with joy, anticipation, and a deep sense of connection to the miracle growing within. It is a time of physical, emotional, and spiritual transformation, as a woman's body nurtures and sustains a new life.

In this book, we recognize the significance of prayer during this sacred period. Prayer allows us to draw closer to our Creator, seeking His guidance, protection, and blessings for both mother and child. It provides a space for reflection, gratitude, and surrender, as we trust in God's plan and His perfect timing.

"Blessings in the Womb" encompasses prayers that cover various aspects of pregnancy, addressing the physical well-being of both mother and child, the emotional challenges and joys, the spiritual growth and connection, and the hopes and dreams for a healthy delivery and post-partum recovery.

Additionally, this prayer handbook includes a special section dedicated to post-partum recovery prayers, recognizing the unique journey of healing and adjustment that follows childbirth. These prayers offer solace, strength, and encouragement during the postpartum period, as mothers navigate the physical and emotional changes while caring for their newborn.

It is our sincere desire that "Blessings in the Womb" becomes a source of inspiration and support for expectant mothers, a companion to turn to during moments of joy, uncertainty, and everything in between. May these prayers bring comfort, peace, and a deepened connection with God throughout the journey of pregnancy and beyond.

As you embark on this extraordinary journey, may you find solace in the words of this prayer handbook, experiencing the boundless blessings that come from nurturing life within, and the immeasurable love of our Heavenly Father who formed each precious child in the womb.

May this book be a beacon of hope, reminding you that you are not alone on this journey. May it serve as a reminder of the incredible privilege and responsibility of motherhood, and may it strengthen your faith, deepen your connection to God, and envelop you in His love and grace.

May "Blessings in the Womb: A Prayer Handbook for Pregnant Women" be a source of inspiration and spiritual nourishment as you embrace the miracles unfolding within you.

May God bless you abundantly as you journey through this sacred season of pregnancy.

HOW TO USE THIS PRAYER BOOK

Congratulations on embarking on this beautiful journey of using "Blessings in the Womb: A Prayer Handbook for Pregnant Women." Here is a guide on how to make the most of this book as you nurture your spiritual connection throughout your pregnancy:

1. Set aside a quiet and comfortable space: Find a peaceful corner in your home where you can retreat, free from distractions. Create an atmosphere that promotes relaxation and tranquility.

2. Choose a specific time each day: Select a time that works best for you to engage in prayer. It could be in the morning, during lunch break, or in the evening. Consistency is key, so aim to establish a daily routine.

3. Read and reflect on one prayer each day: Start with Day 1 and read the prayer provided. Take a moment to reflect on the words, allowing them to sink deep into your heart. Consider how the prayer speaks to your current journey and emotions.

4. Meditate on the accompanying Bible verse: Each prayer is accompanied by a relevant Bible verse. Spend a few moments meditating on the verse, allowing its message to resonate within you. Consider how it relates to your own experiences and offers guidance.

5. Personalize the prayer: After reading the prayer, take a moment to personalize it. Add your own thoughts, feelings, and specific requests. Make it a heartfelt conver-

sation with God, pouring out your joys, concerns, and hopes.

6. Repeat the prayer throughout the day: Whenever you feel the need for reassurance, encouragement, or connection, revisit the prayer of the day. Repeat it in your mind or speak it aloud. Let it become a constant companion, reminding you of God's presence.

7. Continue the cycle for 31 days: Follow the daily prayers for the entire duration of your pregnancy. Allow each prayer to guide and inspire you as you navigate the various stages and emotions of this miraculous journey. You should pray each prayer according to the date of that day. From day 1 of the month to the last day of the month

8. Transition to post-partum recovery prayers after delivery: Once you have given birth, you can begin the section dedicated to post-partum recovery prayers. These prayers will offer solace, healing, and strength during the postpartum period.

9. Confess by faith believing the daily faith confession and you would have a strong faith all through the period of pregnancy and the words you have confessed will become reality in your life

Remember, this book is a tool to deepen your spiritual connection with God during your pregnancy. It is not about rigid adherence or perfect execution but rather about creating moments of intimacy with the Divine. Allow the prayers to become a source of comfort, guidance, and peace as you prepare to welcome your child into the world.

May your journey through pregnancy be blessed with abundant love, grace, and spiritual growth. May this prayer handbook serve as a constant reminder of God's presence and the power of prayer in nurturing your soul.

MONDAYS FAITH CONFESSION

1. I declare that my pregnancy is a blessing from God, and I am filled with gratitude for this precious gift of life. I have faith that God is watching over me and my unborn child, protecting us and guiding us every step of the way.

2. I confess that I am fearfully and wonderfully made, and my body is designed to nurture and sustain a new life. I trust in God's divine plan for my pregnancy, knowing that He has equipped me with the strength and abilities to carry and deliver a healthy baby.

3. I declare that throughout my pregnancy, I will experience a peace that surpasses all understanding. I cast all my anxieties and worries upon the Lord, knowing that He cares for me and my unborn child.

4. I confess that my unborn child is blessed and favored by God. I speak words of love, joy, and positivity over my baby, believing that he/she is fearfully and wonderfully made. I declare that my child will grow and develop according to God's perfect plan.

5. I confess that I am surrounded by a loving and supportive community. I am grateful for my family, friends, and healthcare providers who are there to provide encouragement, assistance, and prayers throughout my pregnancy journey.

6. I declare that I will take care of my physical, emotional, and spiritual well-being during this pregnancy. I will nourish my body with wholesome food, engage in gentle

exercises, and prioritize rest and relaxation. I will seek God's presence daily through prayer, meditation, and reading His Word.

7. I confess that I will walk in faith and not in fear throughout my pregnancy. I trust in God's promises and His unfailing love for me and my baby. I surrender all my worries and concerns to Him, knowing that He is in control.

TUESDAYS FAITH CONFESSION

1. I declare that my pregnancy is a testimony of God's faithfulness and goodness. I am grateful for the miracle of life growing within me and I trust in God's plan and purpose for this child.

2. I confess that God's protection surrounds me and my unborn child. I am covered by His love and grace, and no weapon formed against us shall prosper. I trust in His divine shield of safety and deliverance.

3. I declare that my body is a temple of the Holy Spirit, and I will honor it by making healthy choices for myself and my baby. I will nourish myself with nutritious food, exercise regularly, and rest when needed. I trust that God will strengthen and sustain me throughout this journey.

4. I confess that God's peace fills my heart and mind, dispelling any anxiety or fear. I choose to focus on His promises and trust that He will provide all that I need for a healthy and safe pregnancy. I surrender my worries and concerns to Him, knowing that He is in control.

5. I declare that my unborn child is fearfully and wonderfully made. I speak words of life, health, and wholeness over my baby, believing that God's divine purpose will be fulfilled in his/her life.

6. I confess that I am not alone in this journey. God is with me every step of the way, and He will never leave me nor forsake me. I trust in His guidance and provision, knowing that He will lead me through this pregnancy

with wisdom and grace.

7. I declare that I will walk in faith and not in fear. I choose
   to trust in God's perfect timing and plan for the delivery
   of my baby. I surrender any worries or concerns about
   the labor and delivery process, knowing that God is in
   control and He will give me the strength and courage I
   need.

8. I confess that my body is strong and capable. I trust
   in God's design for childbirth and believe that He will
   empower me for a smooth and successful delivery. I release any fears or doubts and embrace the joy and excitement of bringing new life into the world.

WEDNESDAYS FAITH CONFESSION

1. I declare that my pregnancy is a season of hope and anticipation. I rejoice in the miracle of life growing within me and I trust in God's perfect timing for the arrival of my baby.

2. I confess that God's grace is abundant in my life. He has chosen me to be a vessel for this precious child, and I am honored to carry this divine assignment. I embrace the challenges and joys of pregnancy, knowing that God will sustain me through it all.

3. I declare that my body is strong and healthy. I choose to prioritize self-care and make choices that promote the well-being of myself and my baby. I trust that God's healing power is at work in every cell of my body, bringing forth health and vitality.

4. I confess that my baby is fearfully and wonderfully made. Each day, my child grows and develops according to God's perfect plan. I speak words of life and blessing over my baby, declaring that he/she is destined for greatness and purpose.

5. I declare that God's peace guards my heart and mind during this pregnancy. I release any worries or anxieties to Him, knowing that He is in control. I choose to focus on His promises and trust that He will provide for every need.

6. I confess that I am surrounded by a loving supportive people. My family, friends, and healthcare providers

stand with me in prayer and encouragement. I am grateful for their presence in my life and their unwavering support throughout this journey.

7. I declare that my pregnancy is a testimony of God's faithfulness. I trust in His unfailing love and believe that He will carry me through any challenges or uncertainties that may arise. I surrender my fears and doubts to Him, knowing that He is my rock and refuge.

8. I confess that I will walk in faith and not in fear. I choose to trust in God's promises and His divine plan for my life and the life of my unborn child. I lean on His strength and guidance, knowing that He will lead me on this journey with wisdom and grace.

THURSDAYS FAITH CONFESSION

1. I declare that my pregnancy is a season of joy and anticipation. I am grateful for the gift of life within me and I embrace the journey that lies ahead. I trust in God's perfect timing and plan for the arrival of my baby.

2. I confess that God's presence is with me every step of the way. He is my comforter, my guide, and my strength. I lean on His everlasting arms, knowing that He will carry me through this pregnancy with love and grace.

3. I declare that my body is fearfully and wonderfully made. It is designed to nurture and sustain the life of my baby. I choose to honor and respect my body by making healthy choices and caring for myself and my baby.

4. I confess that my baby is a blessing from God. I speak words of life and destiny over my child, believing that he/she is fearfully and wonderfully made. I declare that my baby will walk in the purpose and calling that God has for his/her life.

5. I declare that my pregnancy is a season of peace and calm. I release any worries or anxieties to God, knowing that He holds me and my baby in the palm of His hand. I choose to rest in His presence and trust in His provision.

6. I confess that God's plans for me and my baby are good. I believe that He will provide everything we need for a healthy and safe pregnancy. I surrender my fears and uncertainties to Him, knowing that He is in control.

7. I declare that my pregnancy is surrounded by love and support. I am grateful for my spouse, family, and friends

who walk alongside me on this journey. I receive their prayers, encouragement, and practical help with open arms. I confess that I will walk in faith and not in fear. I choose to trust in God's promises and His faithfulness. I believe that He will carry me through any challenges or obstacles that may arise during my pregnancy. I place my hope and confidence in Him.

FRIDAYS FAITH CONFESSION

1. I declare that my pregnancy is a testimony of God's faithfulness and grace. I am humbled and grateful for the privilege to carry a new life within me. I trust in His divine plan and purpose for this child.

2. I confess that God's hand is upon me and my unborn baby. He watches over us and protects us from harm. I surrender my fears and worries to Him, knowing that He is in control and He will guide us through this journey.

3. I declare that my body is a temple of the Holy Spirit. I choose to honor God by taking care of myself physically, emotionally, and spiritually during this pregnancy. I will eat nourishing food, engage in gentle exercise, and seek His presence through prayer and meditation.

4. I confess that my baby is fearfully and wonderfully made. I speak words of blessing and life over my child, believing that God has a special purpose for him/her. I pray for the development and growth of my baby, that he/she will be healthy and strong.

5. I declare that my pregnancy is a season of joy and celebration. I choose to focus on the positive aspects and cherish each milestone. I will not be overwhelmed by the challenges but will embrace the journey with gratitude and hope.

6. I confess that God's peace reigns in my heart and mind. I release any anxiety or worry to Him, knowing that He is my refuge and strength. I choose to trust in His unfailing love and believe that He will provide all that I need for a

successful pregnancy.

7. I declare that I am surrounded by a supportive community. I am grateful for my spouse, family, and friends who offer their love, prayers, and practical help. I receive their support with gratitude and open arms.

8. I confess that I will walk in faith and not in fear. I trust in God's promises and His faithfulness. I believe that He will carry me through any challenges or uncertainties that may arise. I place my confidence in His guidance and provision.

SATURDAYS FAITH CONFESSION

1. I declare that my pregnancy is a season of hope and expectation. I am filled with awe and wonder at the miracle of life growing within me. I trust in God's plan and purpose for this child and for myself as a mother.

2. I confess that God's hand is upon me and my unborn baby. He knows us intimately and He is intricately involved in every stage of development. I rest in His loving care and protection.

3. I declare that my body is a vessel of life. I am strong and capable, and I embrace the changes and challenges that come with pregnancy. I trust in God's wisdom and design, knowing that He has equipped me for this journey.

4. I confess that my baby is fearfully and wonderfully made. I speak words of love, health, and destiny over my child, believing that God has great plans for his/her life. I pray for the formation of every part of my baby's body, that he/she will be whole and complete.

5. I declare that my pregnancy is a time of peace and tranquility. I release any stress or anxiety to God, knowing that He holds the future in His hands. I choose to rest in His presence and trust in His perfect timing.

6. I confess that God's provision is abundant in my life. He supplies all my needs, both physical and emotional. I surrender any worries about finances or resources to Him, knowing that He is my provider.

7. I declare that I am surrounded by a loving supportive

people. I am grateful for my spouse, family, and friends who offer their love, encouragement, and prayers. I receive their support with gratitude and open arms.

8. I confess that I will walk in faith and not in fear. I choose to trust in God's promises and His faithfulness. I believe that He will guide me through every step of this journey and that His grace is more than sufficient for all my needs.

SUNDAYS FAITH CONFESSION

1. I declare that my pregnancy is a season of divine purpose. God has entrusted me with the privilege of nurturing and bringing forth new life. I embrace this calling with humility and gratitude.

2. I confess that God's wisdom and guidance are available to me. I seek His direction and understanding as I make decisions regarding my health, the well-being of my baby, and the choices I make during this pregnancy.

3. I declare that my body is a temple of the Holy Spirit. I treat it with respect and care, knowing that I am a steward of this gift of life. I choose to nourish myself with healthy food, exercise, rest, and self-care.

4. I confess that my baby is a gift from God. I speak words of blessing, love, and purpose over my child, believing that he/she is fearfully and wonderfully made. I pray for God's protection and guidance throughout his/her life.

5. I declare that my pregnancy is a time of joy and celebration. I choose to focus on the miracle of life and the blessings that come with motherhood. I rejoice in each kick, each flutter, and each milestone reached.

6. I confess that God's peace fills my heart and mind. I release any anxiety or worry to Him, knowing that He is in control. I trust in His faithfulness and provision, knowing that He will meet all my needs.

7. I declare that I am surrounded by a supportive community. I am grateful for my spouse, family, friends, and healthcare providers who walk alongside me during this

journey. I receive their love, prayers, and assistance with gratitude.

8. I confess that I will walk in faith and not in fear. I trust in God's promises and His unfailing love. I believe that He is with me every step of the way, guiding me, and empowering me to be the mother He has called me to be.

DAY 1: PRAYERS FOR THE MIRACLE OF LIFE

1. Heavenly Father, I thank You for the gift of life within me. I pray that You will sustain and protect this precious child. 'For you created my inmost being; you knit me together in my mother's womb' (Psalm 139:13).

2. Lord, as I embark on this journey of motherhood, I ask for Your guidance and wisdom. Grant me patience and strength to face the challenges ahead. 'Trust in the Lord with all your heart, and do not lean on your own understanding' (Proverbs 3:5).

3. Gracious God, I pray for good health and well-being for both me and my unborn baby. May Your healing touch be upon us. 'For I will restore health to you, and your wounds I will heal, declares the Lord' (Jeremiah 30:17).

4. Dear Lord, I surrender my fears and worries about this pregnancy into Your loving hands. Fill my heart with peace and assurance, knowing that You are in control. 'Do not be anxious about anything, but in everything by prayer and supplication with thanksgiving let your requests be made known to God' (Philippians 4:6).

5. Gracious Father, I pray for the physical strength and endurance to carry this child. Strengthen my body and grant me the energy I need. 'But they who wait for the Lord shall renew their strength; they shall mount up with wings like eagles; they shall run and not be weary; they shall walk and not faint' (Isaiah 40:31).

6. Loving God, I lift up my hopes and dreams for this baby. May they grow up to know You, love You, and walk in Your ways. 'Train up a child in the way he should go; even when he is old he will not depart from it' (Proverbs 22:6).

7. Heavenly Father, I pray for emotional stability and peace during this time of pregnancy. Help me to find comfort in Your presence and to trust in Your plans. 'You keep him in perfect peace whose mind is stayed on you because he trusts in you' (Isaiah 26:3).

8. Dear Lord, I pray for a strong support system of family and friends during this pregnancy. Surround me with people who will uplift and encourage me. 'Two are better than one, because they have a good reward for their toil' (Ecclesiastes 4:9).

9. Gracious God, I pray for the bond between me and my unborn child to grow stronger each day. May our hearts be connected in love, and may I be a vessel of Your nurturing and unconditional care. 'But you, God, see the trouble of the afflicted; you consider their grief and take it in hand' (Psalm 10:14).

10. Lord, I thank You for the joy and anticipation that this pregnancy brings. Help me to embrace each moment and to be grateful for the miracle of life. 'The Lord has done great things for us, and we are filled with joy' (Psalm 126:3).

DAY 2: PRAYERS FOR HEALTH AND WELLNESS

1. Heavenly Father, I pray for the continued health and well-being of both me and my unborn child. Protect us from any harm or complications during this pregnancy. 'Beloved, I pray that all may go well with you and that you may be in good health, as it goes well with your soul' (3 John 1:2).

2. Lord, I lift up my concerns and fears about any potential genetic or prenatal conditions. Grant me peace of mind and trust in Your plan. 'Fear not, for I am with you; be not dismayed, for I am your God; I will strengthen you, I will help you, I will uphold you with my righteous right hand' (Isaiah 41:10).

3. Gracious God, I pray for the development and growth of my baby's body, mind, and spirit. May every part of their being be formed perfectly according to Your divine design. 'For you formed my inward parts; you knitted me together in my mother's womb' (Psalm 139:13).

4. Dear Lord, I ask for Your guidance in making choices that promote a healthy pregnancy. Grant me wisdom in nourishing my body and practicing self-care. 'Or do you not know that your body is a temple of the Holy Spirit within you, whom you have from God? You are not your own' (1 Corinthians 6:19).

5. Loving Father, I pray for relief from any discomfort or physical challenges I may experience during this preg-

nancy. Grant me strength to endure and a sense of peace in the midst of it all. 'Come to me, all who labor and are heavy laden, and I will give you rest' (Matthew 11:28).

6. Heavenly Father, I thank You for the medical professionals who are caring for me and my baby. Grant them wisdom, knowledge, and skill in providing the best care possible. 'For I will restore health to you, and your wounds I will heal, declares the Lord' (Jeremiah 30:17).

7. Lord, I pray for protection from any external threats or harmful influences that may impact the well-being of my unborn child. Surround us with Your divine shield of love and security. 'But the Lord is faithful. He will establish you and guard you against the evil one' (2 Thessalonians 3:3).

8. Gracious God, I ask for strength and resilience to face any unexpected challenges that may arise during this pregnancy. Help me to trust in Your plan and to have confidence in Your provision. 'I can do all things through him who strengthens me' (Philippians 4:13).

9. Dear Lord, I pray for sound sleep and restful nights throughout this pregnancy. Grant me the rejuvenation I need to face each day with energy and joy. 'In peace I will both lie down and sleep; for you alone, O Lord, make me dwell in safety' (Psalm 4:8).

10. Loving Father, I thank You for the gift of life growing within me. Help me to appreciate and cherish this incredible journey of pregnancy. Fill my heart with gratitude and awe for the miracle of creation. 'I praise you,

for I am fearfully and wonderfully made. Wonderful are your works; my soul knows it very well' (Psalm 139:14).

DAY 3: PRAYERS FOR EMOTIONAL WELL-BEING

1. Heavenly Father, I pray for emotional stability and peace during this time of pregnancy. Help me to navigate the hormonal changes and emotional ups and downs with grace and resilience. 'The Lord is near to the broken-hearted and saves the crushed in spirit' (Psalm 34:18).

2. Lord, I lift up any anxieties or worries that weigh heavy on my heart. Grant me Your peace that surpasses all understanding and calm my restless thoughts. 'Do not be anxious about anything, but in everything by prayer and supplication with thanksgiving let your requests be made known to God' (Philippians 4:6).

3. Gracious God, I pray for a positive and joyful mindset throughout this pregnancy. Fill me with hope, optimism, and gratitude for the blessings that come with carrying new life. 'May the God of hope fill you with all joy and peace in believing, so that by the power of the Holy Spirit you may abound in hope' (Romans 15:13).

4. Dear Lord, I ask for Your comfort and strength during moments of pregnancy-related discomfort or pain. Ease my physical discomfort and grant me relief. 'Blessed be the God and Father of our Lord Jesus Christ, the Father of mercies and God of all comfort' (2 Corinthians 1:3).

5. Loving Father, I pray for a healthy and balanced emotional connection with my unborn child. Help me to bond deeply with them, even before their arrival. 'For you

formed my inward parts; you knitted me together in my mother's womb' (Psalm 139:13).

6. Heavenly Father, I surrender my fears of inadequacy and doubt as I step into the role of a mother. Fill me with confidence and remind me that You have equipped me for this journey. 'I can do all things through him who strengthens me' (Philippians 4:13).

7. Lord, I pray for moments of stillness and reflection during this busy time. Help me to find solace in Your presence and to listen to Your gentle whispers. 'Be still, and know that I am God' (Psalm 46:10).

8. Gracious God, I ask for discernment and wisdom as I make important decisions regarding my health and the well-being of my baby. Guide me in choosing what is best for us. 'If any of you lacks wisdom, let him ask God, who gives generously to all without reproach, and it will be given him' (James 1:5).

9. Dear Lord, I pray for protection over my emotions and thoughts, guarding them from negativity and harmful influences. Fill my mind with positivity, gratitude, and love. 'Finally, brothers, whatever is true, whatever is honorable, whatever is just, whatever is pure, whatever is lovely, whatever is commendable, if there is any excellence, if there is anything worthy of praise, think about these things' (Philippians 4:8).

10. Loving Father, I thank You for the gift of emotional resilience. Help me to bounce back from challenging moments and to find strength in Your unfailing love. 'The Lord is my strength and my shield; in him my heart

trusts, and I am helped; my heart exults, and with my song, I give thanks to him' (Psalm 28:7).

DAY 4: PRAYERS FOR BONDING AND CONNECTION

1. Heavenly Father, I pray for a deep and unbreakable bond between me and my unborn child. May our love for each other grow with each passing day. 'So we, though many, are one body in Christ, and individually members one of another' (Romans 12:5).

2. Lord, I ask for moments of connection and communication with my baby. Help me to cherish the tiny kicks and movements as a reminder of the miracle of life within me. 'For you formed my inward parts; you knitted me together in my mother's womb' (Psalm 139:13).

3. Gracious God, I pray for a nurturing and loving environment for my baby to thrive in. May our home be filled with Your peace, joy, and unconditional love. 'Beloved, let us love one another, for love is from God, and whoever loves has been born of God and knows God' (1 John 4:7).

4. Dear Lord, I surrender any fears or doubts I may have about my ability to be a loving and caring mother. Fill me with confidence and remind me that You have entrusted me with this precious gift. 'I can do all things through him who strengthens me' (Philippians 4:13).

5. Loving Father, I pray for patience and understanding as I navigate the changes and challenges of pregnancy. Help me to be kind to myself and to embrace the process with grace. 'Put on then, as God's chosen ones,

holy and beloved, compassionate hearts, kindness, humility, meekness, and patience' (Colossians 3:12).

6. Heavenly Father, I ask for wisdom in forming a strong support system during this pregnancy. Surround me with loved ones who will uplift, encourage, and journey alongside me. 'Two are better than one, because they have a good reward for their toil' (Ecclesiastes 4:9).

7. Lord, I pray for the ability to listen and respond to the needs of my unborn child. Help me to attune to their presence and to be attentive to their well-being. 'My sheep hear my voice, and I know them, and they follow me' (John 10:27).

8. Gracious God, I lift up any barriers or distractions that hinder the bonding process. Help me to be fully present and engaged with my baby, cherishing each moment we spend together. 'Be still, and know that I am God' (Psalm 46:10).

9. Dear Lord, I ask for forgiveness for any times when I have neglected or taken for granted the gift of life within me. Help me to honor and appreciate this miracle with awe and reverence. 'Children are a heritage from the Lord, offspring a reward from him' (Psalm 127:3).

10. Loving Father, I thank You for the privilege of being a mother. May my love for my child reflect Your unconditional love and grace. 'And above all these put on love, which binds everything together in perfect harmony' (Colossians 3:14).

DAY 5: PRAYERS FOR WISDOM AND GUIDANCE

1. Heavenly Father, I pray for wisdom and discernment as I make decisions regarding my pregnancy, childbirth, and parenting. Guide me in choosing what is best for me and my baby. 'If any of you lacks wisdom, let him ask God, who gives generously to all without reproach, and it will be given him' (James 1:5).

2. Lord, I surrender my worries and uncertainties about the future of my child. Fill me with trust and confidence in Your divine plan. 'For I know the plans I have for you, declares the Lord, plans for welfare and not for evil, to give you a future and a hope' (Jeremiah 29:11).

3. Gracious God, I pray for guidance in nurturing and raising my child in a way that pleases You. Help me to be an example of Your love, grace, and righteousness. 'Train up a child in the way he should go; even when he is old he will not depart from it' (Proverbs 22:6).

4. Dear Lord, I ask for insight and understanding as I learn about the various stages of pregnancy and the development of my baby. Grant me the knowledge to care for them well. 'For the Lord gives wisdom; from his mouth come knowledge and understanding' (Proverbs 2:6).

5. Loving Father, I pray for discernment in making choices that promote a healthy lifestyle for myself and my unborn child. Help me to prioritize their well-being in all aspects. 'Or do you not know that your body is a temple

of the Holy Spirit within you, whom you have from God? You are not your own' (1 Corinthians 6:19).

6. Heavenly Father, I seek Your guidance in finding the right healthcare providers who will support and care for me and my baby throughout this pregnancy. Lead me to skilled professionals who align with Your plans. 'Commit your work to the Lord, and your plans will be established' (Proverbs 16:3).

7. Lord, I pray for wisdom in preparing for the arrival of my baby. Help me to make practical and thoughtful decisions in creating a safe and welcoming environment. 'By wisdom a house is built, and by understanding, it is established' (Proverbs 24:3).

8. Gracious God, I ask for Your wisdom and guidance in choosing a name for my child. May their name carry meaning and significance that aligns with Your purpose for their life. 'The name of the Lord is a strong tower; the righteous man runs into it and is safe' (Proverbs 18:10).

9. Dear Lord, I surrender my desires and expectations for my child's future into Your hands. Grant me the wisdom to support and encourage them in discovering their unique gifts and talents. 'For we are his workmanship, created in Christ Jesus for good works, which God prepared beforehand, that we should walk in them' (Ephesians 2:10).

10. Loving Father, I thank You for the promise of Your Holy Spirit, who guides and teaches me in all things. Help me to rely on Your wisdom and direction every step of this journey. 'But the Helper, the Holy Spirit, whom the

Father will send in my name, he will teach you all things and bring to your remembrance all that I have said to you' (John 14:26).

DAY 6: PRAYERS FOR PATIENCE AND TRUST

1. Heavenly Father, I pray for an abundance of patience as I navigate the journey of pregnancy. Help me to embrace each day with a calm and trusting heart. 'But if we hope for what we do not see, we wait for it with patience' (Romans 8:25).

2. Lord, I surrender my worries and anxieties about the timing and process of childbirth. Fill me with trust in Your perfect timing and the strength to endure. 'Trust in the Lord with all your heart, and do not lean on your own understanding' (Proverbs 3:5).

3. Gracious God, I ask for patience and understanding in dealing with the physical discomforts and limitations of pregnancy. Grant me resilience and the ability to find joy in the midst of challenges. 'May you be strengthened with all power, according to his glorious might, for all endurance and patience with joy' (Colossians 1:11).

4. Dear Lord, I pray for patience and grace in my relationships during this pregnancy. Help me to extend kindness and understanding to those around me, even in moments of heightened emotions. 'Put on then, as God's chosen ones, holy and beloved, compassionate hearts, kindness, humility, meekness, and patience' (Colossians 3:12).

5. Loving Father, I ask for patience and wisdom in preparing for the arrival of my baby. Help me to embrace the

process and not be overwhelmed by the tasks at hand. 'And let us not grow weary of doing good, for in due season we will reap if we do not give up' (Galatians 6:9).

6. Heavenly Father, I pray for patience and trust as I wait for the fulfillment of Your promises for my child's life. Give me confidence that Your plans are good and that You will be faithful to fulfill them. 'The Lord is not slow to fulfill his promise as some count slowness but is patient toward you' (2 Peter 3:9).

7. Lord, I ask for patience in moments of uncertainty or fear. Help me to lean on Your strength and trust that You are with me through every step of this journey. 'Have I not commanded you? Be strong and courageous. Do not be frightened, and do not be dismayed, for the Lord your God is with you wherever you go' (Joshua 1:9).

8. Gracious God, I pray for patience and flexibility in adapting to the changes that come with pregnancy. Help me to embrace the unknown and find peace in surrendering to Your plans. 'For I know the plans I have for you, declares the Lord, plans for welfare and not for evil, to give you a future and a hope' (Jeremiah 29:11).

9. Dear Lord, I surrender my impatience and the desire for control. Fill me with a spirit of surrender and acceptance, knowing that You are in control of all things. 'Commit your way to the Lord; trust in him, and he will act' (Psalm 37:5).

10. Loving Father, I thank You for the opportunity to cultivate patience and trust through this pregnancy. Help me to grow in these virtues and rely on Your guidance

in every moment. 'May the God of endurance and encouragement grant you to live in such harmony with one another, in accord with Christ Jesus' (Romans 15:5).

DAY 7: PRAYERS FOR PROTECTION AND SAFETY

1. Heavenly Father, I pray for Your divine protection over me and my unborn child. Guard us from harm and surround us with Your angels of protection. 'The Lord will keep you from all evil; he will keep your life' (Psalm 121:7).

2. Lord, I surrender any fears or anxieties I have about the well-being and safety of my baby. Fill me with faith and assurance that You are watching over them. 'But the Lord is faithful. He will establish you and guard you against the evil one' (2 Thessalonians 3:3).

3. Gracious God, I pray for the safety and health of my baby throughout this pregnancy. May they grow and develop according to Your perfect design. 'For you formed my inward parts; you knitted me together in my mother's womb' (Psalm 139:13).

4. Dear Lord, I ask for Your protection during labor and delivery. Guide the hands of the medical professionals attending to me and grant me a safe and smooth childbirth experience. 'Fear not, for I am with you; be not dismayed, for I am your God; I will strengthen you, I will help you, I will uphold you with my righteous right hand' (Isaiah 41:10).

5. Loving Father, I pray for protection from any complications or challenges that may arise during this pregnancy. Help me to trust in Your power to overcome any ob-

stacles. 'The name of the Lord is a strong tower; the righteous man runs into it and is safe' (Proverbs 18:10).

6. Heavenly Father, I ask for Your divine protection over my emotional and mental well-being during this pregnancy. Guard my heart and mind from anxiety and fill me with Your peace. 'And the peace of God, which surpasses all understanding, will guard your hearts and your minds in Christ Jesus' (Philippians 4:7).

7. Lord, I pray for protection from external influences or negative energies that may affect my baby. Surround us with Your shield of love and keep us safe from harm. 'But you, O Lord, are a shield about me, my glory, and the lifter of my head' (Psalm 3:3).

8. Gracious God, I surrender my fears and concerns about the safety of my baby's future. Help me to trust in Your sovereign plan and believe that You hold their future in Your hands. 'For I know the plans I have for you, declares the Lord, plans for welfare and not for evil, to give you a future and a hope' (Jeremiah 29:11).

9. Dear Lord, I ask for protection from stress and worry that may affect my well-being and that of my baby. Grant me peace and serenity as I rest in Your loving care. 'Come to me, all who labor and are heavy laden, and I will give you rest' (Matthew 11:28).

10. Loving Father, I thank You for Your unwavering protection and faithfulness. Help me to trust in Your constant presence and find comfort in knowing that You are always watching over us. 'The Lord is my rock and my fortress and my deliverer, my God, my rock, in whom I

take refuge, my shield, and the horn of my salvation, my stronghold' (Psalm 18:2).

DAY 8: PRAYERS FOR STRENGTH AND ENDURANCE

1. Heavenly Father, I pray for physical strength and endurance as my body undergoes the changes of pregnancy. Grant me the energy to face each day with vitality and resilience. 'I can do all things through him who strengthens me' (Philippians 4:13).

2. Lord, I surrender my weariness and fatigue to You. Renew my strength and refresh my spirit when I feel overwhelmed. 'He gives power to the faint, and to him who has no might he increases strength' (Isaiah 40:29).

3. Gracious God, I pray for emotional and mental strength during this pregnancy. Help me to remain grounded in Your peace and find solace in Your presence. 'The Lord is my strength and my shield; in him my heart trusts, and I am helped' (Psalm 28:7).

4. Dear Lord, I ask for spiritual strength to nourish and strengthen my faith throughout this journey. May I find comfort and guidance in Your Word and in communion with You. 'But they who wait for the Lord shall renew their strength; they shall mount up with wings like eagles; they shall run and not be weary; they shall walk and not faint' (Isaiah 40:31).

5. Loving Father, I pray for the strength to embrace the challenges and sacrifices that come with motherhood. Grant me the courage to persevere and the wisdom to make selfless choices for the well-being of my child. 'Be

strong, and let your heart take courage, all you who wait for the Lord!' (Psalm 31:24).

6. Heavenly Father, I ask for strength and patience in dealing with any discomforts or pains associated with pregnancy. Help me to endure with grace, knowing that this journey is temporary and leads to the miracle of new life. 'And after you have suffered a little while, the God of all grace, who has called you to his eternal glory in Christ, will himself restore, confirm, strengthen, and establish you' (1 Peter 5:10).

7. Lord, I pray for strength and perseverance in facing any complications or medical challenges that may arise during this pregnancy. Grant me the courage to trust in Your healing power and the strength to overcome obstacles. 'The Lord is my strength and my song; he has become my salvation' (Psalm 118:14).

8. Gracious God, I surrender my fears and insecurities about my ability to be a strong and capable mother. Fill me with confidence and remind me that You equip me for every task You place before me. 'For God gave us a spirit not of fear but of power and love and self-control' (2 Timothy 1:7).

9. Dear Lord, I ask for strength to navigate the emotional ups and downs of pregnancy. Help me to embrace the joys and challenges with resilience and a steadfast spirit. 'But he said to me, 'My grace is sufficient for you, for my power is made perfect in weakness.' Therefore I will boast all the more gladly of my weaknesses, so that the power of Christ may rest upon me' (2 Corinthians 12:9).

10. Loving Father, I thank You for being my ultimate source of strength. Help me to rely on You in times of weakness and to find comfort in Your presence. 'The Lord is my strength and my song; he has become my salvation' (Psalm 118:14).

DAY 9: PRAYERS FOR HEALTHY DEVELOPMENT

1. Heavenly Father, I pray for the healthy development of my unborn child. May every organ, every cell, and every system form according to Your perfect design. 'For you formed my inward parts; you knitted me together in my mother's womb' (Psalm 139:13).

2. Lord, I surrender any concerns or fears I have about the development of my baby. Fill me with faith and confidence that You are intricately involved in their growth and that You hold their future in Your hands. 'Before I formed you in the womb, I knew you' (Jeremiah 1:5).

3. Gracious God, I pray for the protection of my baby's physical and mental well-being during this critical stage of development. Shield them from any harm or abnormalities, and grant them strength and vitality. 'May you be strengthened with all power, according to his glorious might' (Colossians 1:11).

4. Dear Lord, I ask for the proper formation and growth of my baby's bones, muscles, and tissues. Guide their development so they may be strong and healthy. 'You knit me together in my mother's womb' (Psalm 139:13).

5. Loving Father, I pray for the development of my baby's senses. May their eyes see the beauty of Your creation, their ears hear the melodies of life, and their senses be attuned to the world around them. 'I praise you, for I am fearfully and wonderfully made' (Psalm 139:14).

6. Heavenly Father, I pray for the healthy development of my baby's brain and nervous system. May their mind be sharp, their intellect be curious, and their mental faculties be well-formed. 'For God gave us a spirit not of fear but of power and love and self-control' (2 Timothy 1:7).

7. Lord, I pray for the proper development of my baby's heart and circulatory system. May their heartbeat strong and steady, and may their blood flow be healthy and nourishing. 'Create in me a clean heart, O God, and renew a right spirit within me' (Psalm 51:10).

8. Gracious God, I ask for the development of my baby's respiratory system. May their lungs form and mature so they can breathe the breath of life with ease. 'Then the Lord God formed the man of dust from the ground and breathed into his nostrils the breath of life, and the man became a living creature' (Genesis 2:7).

9. Dear Lord, I pray for the healthy development of my baby's digestive system. May their body assimilate nutrients and eliminate waste effectively, promoting growth and vitality. 'So whether you eat or drink, or whatever you do, do all to the glory of God' (1 Corinthians 10:31).

10. Loving Father, I thank You for the miraculous process of life unfolding within me. Help me to cherish and nurture this precious gift, trusting in Your wisdom and provision for the optimal development of my baby. 'For you formed my inward parts; you knitted me together in my mother's womb' (Psalm 139:13).

DAY 10: PRAYERS FOR SPIRITUAL NURTURING

1. Heavenly Father, I pray for the spiritual well-being and growth of my unborn child. May their heart be open to Your love and their spirit be attuned to Your presence. 'And this is eternal life, that they know you, the only true God, and Jesus Christ whom you have sent' (John 17:3).

2. Lord, I surrender my desires and plans for my child's future to You. May they grow to know and love You deeply, walking in Your ways and fulfilling the purpose You have for their life. 'Commit your work to the Lord, and your plans will be established' (Proverbs 16:3).

3. Gracious God, I pray for spiritual protection over my baby. Guard their heart and mind from worldly influences and lead them in the paths of righteousness. 'Blessed are those who keep his testimonies, who seek him with their whole heart' (Psalm 119:2).

4. Dear Lord, I ask for the nurturing of faith and a love for Your Word in my child's life. May they find comfort, wisdom, and guidance in the Scriptures throughout their journey. 'Your word is a lamp to my feet and a light to my path' (Psalm 119:105).

5. Loving Father, I pray for godly influences and role models in my child's life. Surround them with mentors, teachers, and loved ones who will guide them in their spiritual walk. 'Iron sharpens iron, and one man sharpens another' (Proverbs 27:17).

6. Heavenly Father, I ask for the development of a humble and teachable spirit in my child. May they always be open to Your leading and willing to follow Your ways. 'Humble yourselves before the Lord, and he will exalt you' (James 4:10).

7. Lord, I pray for the gift of discernment in my child's life. May they have the wisdom to distinguish between truth and deception, and to make choices that align with Your will. 'But solid food is for the mature, for those who have their powers of discernment trained by constant practice to distinguish good from evil' (Hebrews 5:14).

8. Gracious God, I ask for a heart of compassion and empathy to be cultivated in my child. May they have a deep love for others and a desire to make a positive impact in the world. 'Put on then, as God's chosen ones, holy and beloved, compassionate hearts, kindness, humility, meekness, and patience' (Colossians 3:12).

9. Dear Lord, I pray for the development of resilience and perseverance in my child's faith. May they hold firm to their beliefs and withstand the challenges and trials that come their way. 'Count it all joy, my brothers, when you meet trials of various kinds' (James 1:2).

10. Loving Father, I thank You for the privilege of nurturing a child's spiritual growth. Help me to lead by example, living out a genuine faith that inspires and encourages my child to follow You wholeheartedly. 'Train up a child in the way he should go; even when he is old he will not depart from it' (Proverbs 22:6).

DAY 11: PRAYERS FOR EMOTIONAL STABILITY

1. Heavenly Father, I pray for emotional stability and balance during this season of pregnancy. Grant me peace amidst hormonal changes and help me to navigate the ups and downs with grace. 'The Lord is near to the brokenhearted and saves the crushed in spirit' (Psalm 34:18).

2. Lord, I surrender any feelings of anxiety or overwhelm to You. Fill me with Your calming presence and grant me a sense of tranquility in the midst of uncertainty. 'Do not be anxious about anything, but in everything by prayer and supplication with thanksgiving let your requests be made known to God' (Philippians 4:6).

3. Gracious God, I pray for emotional resilience and strength. Help me to face any emotional challenges with courage and trust in Your unfailing love. 'Have I not commanded you? Be strong and courageous. Do not be frightened, and do not be dismayed, for the Lord your God is with you wherever you go' (Joshua 1:9).

4. Dear Lord, I ask for the ability to process and express my emotions in healthy ways. Guide me to find outlets for my feelings and grant me the wisdom to seek support when needed. 'A friend loves at all times, and a brother is born for adversity' (Proverbs 17:17).

5. Loving Father, I pray for emotional bonding and connection with my unborn child. May our hearts be intertwined

with love and understanding, fostering a strong and nurturing relationship. 'So we, though many, are one body in Christ, and individually members one of another' (Romans 12:5).

6. Heavenly Father, I ask for emotional healing from any past hurts or traumas that may affect my well-being during pregnancy. Pour out Your comforting and restoring grace upon my heart. 'He heals the brokenhearted and binds up their wounds' (Psalm 147:3).

7. Lord, I pray for emotional stability and harmony within my relationships during this season. Grant me the ability to communicate with love and understanding, fostering healthy connections with my loved ones. 'A soft answer turns away wrath, but a harsh word stirs up anger' (Proverbs 15:1).

8. Gracious God, I surrender any feelings of guilt or inadequacy to You. Help me to embrace my emotions without judgment and to extend grace to myself as I navigate the challenges of pregnancy. 'There is therefore now no condemnation for those who are in Christ Jesus' (Romans 8:1).

9. Dear Lord, I pray for a spirit of joy and gratitude to permeate my heart throughout this pregnancy. Help me to focus on the blessings and to cultivate a positive mindset. 'Rejoice always, pray without ceasing, give thanks in all circumstances; for this is the will of God in Christ Jesus for you' (1 Thessalonians 5:16-18).

10. Loving Father, I thank You for the gift of emotions and the depth they add to our human experience. Help me to

surrender my emotions to You, seeking Your guidance and strength to navigate them with wisdom and grace. 'For you, O Lord, have made me glad by your work; at the works of your hands I sing for joy' (Psalm 92:4).

DAY 12: PRAYERS FOR REST AND RENEWAL

1. Heavenly Father, I come before You seeking rest and renewal for my body, mind, and spirit. Grant me the ability to find moments of true rest amidst the busyness of pregnancy. 'Come to me, all who labor and are heavy laden, and I will give you rest' (Matthew 11:28).

2. Lord, I surrender any worries or anxieties that may disrupt my sleep. Grant me peaceful and restorative rest each night, allowing my body to rejuvenate. 'In peace I will both lie down and sleep; for you alone, O Lord, make me dwell in safety' (Psalm 4:8).

3. Gracious God, I pray for physical strength and vitality during this season. Help me to listen to my body's cues and to care for it with proper nutrition, exercise, and rest. 'Do you not know that your body is a temple of the Holy Spirit within you, whom you have from God?' (1 Corinthians 6:19).

4. Dear Lord, I ask for mental and emotional rest amidst the thoughts and concerns that arise during pregnancy. Grant me clarity of mind and the ability to surrender worries to Your loving care. 'Be still, and know that I am God' (Psalm 46:10).

5. Loving Father, I pray for moments of spiritual refreshing and renewal. May I find solace in Your presence and draw near to You in times of prayer and meditation. 'But they who wait for the Lord shall renew their strength; they

shall mount up with wings like eagles' (Isaiah 40:31).

6. Heavenly Father, I ask for the ability to set healthy boundaries and prioritize self-care during pregnancy. Help me to recognize when I need rest and to give myself permission to take time for rejuvenation. 'But Jesus often withdrew to lonely places and prayed' (Luke 5:16).

7. Lord, I pray for a peaceful and nurturing environment that promotes rest and relaxation. May my surroundings be a sanctuary of tranquility where I can find solace and recharge. 'Make me to lie down in green pastures; lead me beside still waters' (Psalm 23:2).

8. Gracious God, I surrender any guilt or pressure to be constantly productive during pregnancy. Help me to embrace the beauty of rest and to trust that it is necessary for the well-being of myself and my baby. 'It is in vain that you rise up early and go late to rest, eating the bread of anxious toil; for he gives to his beloved sleep' (Psalm 127:2).

9. Dear Lord, I pray for moments of leisure and enjoyment during pregnancy. Grant me opportunities to engage in activities that bring me joy and allow me to savor the blessings of this season. 'A joyful heart is good medicine' (Proverbs 17:22).

10. Loving Father, I thank You for the gift of rest and renewal. Help me to embrace these moments as sacred and necessary for my well-being. Fill me with Your peace and restore my energy as I trust in Your provision. 'For I will satisfy the weary soul, and every languishing soul I will replenish' (Jeremiah 31:25).

DAY 13: PRAYERS FOR STRONG SUPPORTIVE PEOPLE

1. Heavenly Father, I thank You for the gift of a supportive community during my pregnancy. Surround me with people who uplift, encourage, and provide practical assistance in this journey. 'Two are better than one, because they have a good reward for their toil' (Ecclesiastes 4:9).

2. Lord, I pray for my spouse or partner as they walk alongside me in this pregnancy. Grant them wisdom, strength, and patience to support me in the physical, emotional, and spiritual aspects of this journey. 'Two are better than one, because they have a good reward for their toil' (Ecclesiastes 4:9).

3. Gracious God, I ask for the presence of caring family members and friends who will offer love, encouragement, and practical help during this season. May their words and actions bring comfort and support. 'Bear one another's burdens, and so fulfill the law of Christ' (Galatians 6:2).

4. Dear Lord, I pray for healthcare professionals who are involved in my prenatal care. Bless them with wisdom, skill, and compassion as they guide and monitor the health of me and my baby. 'May the God of all endurance and encouragement grant you to live in such harmony with one another' (Romans 15:5).

5. Loving Father, I pray for a strong network of fellow ex-

pectant mothers with whom I can share experiences, insights, and encouragement. May we support and uplift one another throughout our pregnancies. 'Therefore encourage one another and build one another up' (1 Thessalonians 5:11).

6. Heavenly Father, I ask for the guidance and support of a trusted mentor or spiritual advisor who can provide wisdom and guidance during this transformative season. May their presence be a source of strength and inspiration. 'Listen to advice and accept instruction, that you may gain wisdom in the future' (Proverbs 19:20).

7. Lord, I pray for a strong online community of resources and support for expectant mothers. May I find encouragement, knowledge, and connection through online platforms that provide valuable insights and shared experiences. 'Iron sharpens iron, and one man sharpens another' (Proverbs 27:17).

8. Gracious God, I ask for the support of local organizations or support groups that cater to the needs of expectant mothers. Guide me to find these valuable resources and to engage with them for guidance and community. 'Two are better than one, because they have a good reward for their toil' (Ecclesiastes 4:9).

9. Dear Lord, I pray for the presence of mentors or role models who have experienced the journey of pregnancy and motherhood. May their wisdom and insight provide guidance and assurance as I navigate this new chapter. 'Listen to advice and accept instruction, that you may gain wisdom in the future' (Proverbs 19:20).

10.   Loving Father, I thank You for the diverse and supportive network of individuals who will walk with me through this pregnancy. Help me to recognize and appreciate their contributions, and may I also be a source of support to others in their journeys. 'Therefore encourage one another and build one another up' (1 Thessalonians 5:11)."

DAY 14: PRAYERS FOR PREPARATION AND ORGANIZATION

1. Heavenly Father, I pray for wisdom and discernment as I prepare for the arrival of my baby. Guide me in making practical decisions and help me to organize my home and life in a way that promotes peace and harmony. 'For God is not a God of confusion but of peace' (1 Corinthians 14:33).

2. Lord, I ask for clarity and focus as I create a plan for the upcoming weeks and months. Grant me the ability to prioritize tasks and responsibilities, and help me to stay organized amidst the busyness of preparing for a new addition to our family. 'Let all things be done decently and in order' (1 Corinthians 14:40).

3. Gracious God, I pray for the provision of the necessary resources and materials needed for the well-being of my baby. Guide me in making wise financial decisions and bless me with the means to provide for their needs. 'And my God will supply every need of yours according to his riches in glory in Christ Jesus' (Philippians 4:19).

4. Dear Lord, I ask for guidance and wisdom as I research and make decisions regarding prenatal classes, childbirth options, and parenting philosophies. Help me to make informed choices that align with my values and desires for my child. 'Trust in the Lord with all your heart, and do not lean on your own understanding' (Proverbs 3:5).

5. Loving Father, I pray for strength and perseverance as I prepare physically for childbirth. Grant me the discipline and motivation to engage in exercises and practices that will contribute to a healthy pregnancy and labor. 'I can do all things through him who strengthens me' (Philippians 4:13).

6. Heavenly Father, I surrender any fears or anxieties about the unknowns of parenthood. Grant me confidence and assurance as I prepare to embrace the joys and challenges of raising a child. 'For God gave us a spirit not of fear but of power and love and self-control' (2 Timothy 1:7).

7. Lord, I ask for the guidance of the Holy Spirit as I make decisions regarding baby names, nursery decor, and other personal choices. May my decisions be infused with love and reflect the unique blessings this child brings to our lives. 'Commit your work to the Lord, and your plans will be established' (Proverbs 16:3).

8. Gracious God, I pray for the strength and resilience to handle the practical tasks of preparing for a baby, such as washing and organizing clothes, setting up the nursery, and gathering essential supplies. May these acts of preparation fill me with joyful anticipation. 'And whatever you do, in word or deed, do everything in the name of the Lord Jesus, giving thanks to God the Father through him' (Colossians 3:17).

9. Dear Lord, I ask for the support and assistance of family and friends as I prepare for the arrival of my baby. Bless them with willing hearts to lend a helping hand and provide guidance and encouragement along the way. 'Two

are better than one, because they have a good reward for their toil' (Ecclesiastes 4:9).

10.   Loving Father, I thank You for the privilege of preparing for the arrival of this precious child. Help me to approach this season with gratitude and excitement, knowing that You are with me every step of the way. 'The Lord your God is in your midst, a mighty one who will save; he will rejoice over you with gladness; he will quiet you by his love; he will exult over you with loud singing' (Zephaniah 3:17).

DAY 15: PRAYERS FOR GOOD HEALTH AND STRENGTH

1. Heavenly Father, I pray for the continued good health and well-being of both myself and my unborn child. Surround us with Your divine protection and grant us strength and vitality throughout this pregnancy journey. 'The Lord is my strength and my shield; in him my heart trusts' (Psalm 28:7).

2. Lord, I surrender any fears or concerns about complications or health issues during pregnancy. I trust in Your sovereignty and ask for Your healing touch to be upon us, shielding us from harm and ensuring a healthy and safe pregnancy. 'Heal me, O Lord, and I shall be healed; save me, and I shall be saved' (Jeremiah 17:14).

3. Gracious God, I pray for the development of my baby's organs, bones, and body systems. May every part of their being grow and form according to Your perfect design. 'For you formed my inward parts; you knitted me together in my mother's womb' (Psalm 139:13).

4. Dear Lord, I ask for strength and endurance as my body undergoes the physical demands of pregnancy. Grant me the energy and resilience to carry this child with grace and to navigate any discomforts that may arise. 'I can do all things through him who strengthens me' (Philippians 4:13).

5. Loving Father, I pray for a strong immune system for both me and my baby. Protect us from illnesses and

infections, and strengthen our bodies to fight off any potential threats. 'He will cover you with his pinions, and under his wings you will find refuge; his faithfulness is a shield and buckler' (Psalm 91:4).

6. Heavenly Father, I lift up any concerns or anxieties I may have regarding genetic or hereditary conditions. I place my trust in Your sovereignty, knowing that You hold the blueprint of my child's life in Your hands. 'For I know the plans I have for you, declares the Lord, plans for welfare and not for evil, to give you a future and a hope' (Jeremiah 29:11).

7. Lord, I pray for healthy growth and weight gain for my baby. May they develop according to Your perfect timing and may their growth be a testament to Your faithfulness and provision. 'Your eyes saw my unformed substance; in your book were written, every one of them, the days that were formed for me, when as yet there was none of them' (Psalm 139:16).

8. Gracious God, I ask for emotional and mental well-being throughout my pregnancy. Guard my mind and heart from anxiety, stress, and negative thoughts. Fill me with peace and serenity as I trust in Your plans for me and my baby. 'The Lord is my rock and my fortress and my deliverer, my God, my rock, in whom I take refuge' (Psalm 18:2).

9. Dear Lord, I pray for the strength to take care of my own physical and mental health during pregnancy. Guide me in making wise choices, nourishing my body with nutritious food, engaging in appropriate exercise, and prioritizing self-care. 'Or do you not know that your body is

a temple of the Holy Spirit within you, whom you have from God?' (1 Corinthians 6:19).

10.   Loving Father, I thank You for the gift of good health and strength. Help me to treasure and appreciate the miracle of life growing within me. May I never take for granted the precious bond between mother and child. 'Children are a heritage from the Lord, the fruit of the womb a reward' (Psalm 127:3).

DAY 16: PRAYERS FOR A SAFE AND SMOOTH DELIVERY

1. Heavenly Father, as the day of delivery approaches, I surrender my fears and anxieties into Your loving hands. Grant me peace and assurance, knowing that You are with me every step of the way. 'Do not fear, for I am with you; do not be dismayed, for I am your God' (Isaiah 41:10).

2. Lord, I pray for a safe and smooth delivery for both me and my baby. I ask for skilled medical professionals and a supportive birthing team who will provide excellent care and guidance throughout the process. 'The Lord is my strength and my song; he has become my salvation' (Psalm 118:14).

3. Gracious God, I pray for the strength and endurance to navigate the challenges of labor. Grant me physical stamina and mental fortitude as I bring forth new life into the world. 'I can do all things through him who strengthens me' (Philippians 4:13).

4. Dear Lord, I surrender my birth plan into Your hands, trusting that Your perfect will shall be done. May the birth of my baby be a testimony to Your faithfulness and a testament to Your sovereign plan. 'Many are the plans in the mind of a man, but it is the purpose of the Lord that will stand' (Proverbs 19:21).

5. Loving Father, I pray for the pain and discomfort of labor to be eased and managed effectively. Grant me peace

amidst the intensity, knowing that You are present and that each contraction brings me closer to the joy of meeting my baby. 'When the righteous cry for help, the Lord hears and delivers them out of all their troubles' (Psalm 34:17).

6. Heavenly Father, I ask for Your divine protection over me and my baby during the delivery process. Guard us from any complications or risks, and let Your angels surround us with their heavenly presence. 'He will cover you with his pinions, and under his wings you will find refuge; his faithfulness is a shield and buckler' (Psalm 91:4).

7. Lord, I pray for a supportive and encouraging birthing environment. Surround me with loving voices, uplifting prayers, and affirming words that will empower me and instill confidence in my ability to birth my baby. 'Therefore encourage one another and build one another up' (1 Thessalonians 5:11).

8. Gracious God, I pray for effective communication and understanding between me and my medical team. May they listen attentively to my needs and desires, and may we work together harmoniously for the well-being of both me and my baby. 'A soft answer turns away wrath, but a harsh word stirs up anger' (Proverbs 15:1).

9. Dear Lord, I ask for Your divine intervention and guidance in any unexpected situations or complications that may arise during labor. Give wisdom to my healthcare providers as they make decisions and guide them in the best course of action. 'The Lord is near to all who call on him, to all who call on him in truth' (Psalm 145:18).

10.   Loving Father, I thank You in advance for the safe delivery of my baby. May the joy and wonder of new life fill the delivery room, and may Your presence bring peace and comfort to all who are present. 'Every good gift and every perfect gift is from above, coming down from the Father of lights' (James 1:17).

DAY 17: PRAYERS FOR HEALTHY DEVELOPMENT IN THE WOMB

1. Heavenly Father, I thank You for the miraculous process of development taking place within me. I pray for the continued growth and formation of every organ, limb, and system of my baby. 'I praise you, for I am fearfully and wonderfully made. Wonderful are your works; my soul knows it very well' (Psalm 139:14).

2. Lord, I pray for the healthy development of my baby's brain and neurological system. May their cognitive abilities, intelligence, and senses develop according to Your perfect design. 'For you formed my inward parts; you knitted me together in my mother's womb' (Psalm 139:13).

3. Gracious God, I lift up prayers for the proper development of my baby's heart and cardiovascular system. May their heart beat strong and steady, and may their blood flow be healthy and nourishing. 'Create in me a clean heart, O God, and renew a right spirit within me' (Psalm 51:10).

4. Dear Lord, I pray for the growth and development of my baby's lungs and respiratory system. May they develop fully and function effectively to sustain life outside the womb. 'The breath of the Almighty gives me life' (Job 33:4).

5. Loving Father, I pray for the formation and growth of my baby's musculoskeletal system. May their bones

strengthen and develop properly, and may their muscles grow and provide support for their growing body. 'He gives strength to the weary and increases the power of the weak' (Isaiah 40:29).

6. Heavenly Father, I lift up prayers for the healthy development of my baby's digestive system. May their stomach, intestines, and other digestive organs form correctly and function optimally to receive nourishment. 'Satisfy us in the morning with your steadfast love, that we may rejoice and be glad all our days' (Psalm 90:14).

7. Lord, I pray for the proper development of my baby's senses—sight, hearing, taste, touch, and smell. May their senses develop fully and allow them to experience the wonders of the world You have created. 'The hearing ear and the seeing eye, the Lord has made them both' (Proverbs 20:12).

8. Gracious God, I pray for the development of my baby's immune system. May it grow strong and resilient, equipping them to fight off infections and diseases. 'For I, the Lord your God, hold your right hand; it is I who say to you, 'Fear not, I am the one who helps you" (Isaiah 41:13).

9. Dear Lord, I pray for the healthy development of my baby's reproductive system. May it form according to Your perfect plan and function properly when the time comes. 'He gives the barren woman a home, making her the joyous mother of children' (Psalm 113:9).

10.   Loving Father, I thank You for the intricate and miraculous development happening within my womb. Help

me to appreciate and marvel at the wonders of life unfolding. 'For you formed my inward parts; you knitted
me together in my mother's womb. I praise you, for I am
fearfully and wonderfully made' (Psalm 139:13-14).

DAY 18: PRAYERS FOR STRENGTH AND PROTECTION AGAINST WEAKNESS AND SICKNESS

1. Heavenly Father, I come before You with a humble heart, seeking Your strength and protection against weakness and sickness during my pregnancy. Fill me with Your divine energy and vitality. 'But he said to me, 'My grace is sufficient for you, for my power is made perfect in weakness' (2 Corinthians 12:9).

2. Lord, I pray for physical strength to endure the demands of pregnancy. Strengthen my body, muscles, and bones, and grant me the stamina to carry this precious life within me. 'The Lord is my strength and my shield; my heart trusts in him, and he helps me' (Psalm 28:7).

3. Gracious God, I ask for protection against common illnesses and infections that can weaken my immune system. Guard me and my baby from any harmful bacteria or viruses, and grant us good health throughout this journey. 'He will cover you with his feathers, and under his wings, you will find refuge; his faithfulness will be your shield and rampart' (Psalm 91:4).

4. Dear Lord, I pray against fatigue and weariness that may weigh me down during pregnancy. Renew my strength each day and restore my energy when I feel depleted. 'Come to me, all who labor and are heavy laden, and I will give you rest' (Matthew 11:28).

5. Loving Father, I ask for protection against pregnancy-re-

lated discomforts and ailments. Shield me from nausea, backaches, headaches, and any other physical challenges that may arise. 'The Lord is my rock, my fortress, and my deliverer; my God is my rock, in whom I take refuge' (Psalm 18:2).

6. Heavenly Father, I pray against anxiety and stress that can weaken both my physical and emotional well-being. Fill me with Your peace and calmness, and help me to cast all my worries upon You. 'Do not be anxious about anything, but in every situation, by prayer and petition, with thanksgiving, present your requests to God' (Philippians 4:6).

7. Lord, I pray for protection against complications or risks that may arise during pregnancy. Guide my medical team, grant them wisdom, and help them to make decisions that promote the well-being of both me and my baby. 'Trust in the Lord with all your heart and lean not on your own understanding' (Proverbs 3:5).

8. Gracious God, I ask for protection against negative thoughts and emotions that can weaken my spirit. Guard my heart and mind, and fill me with positivity, hope, and resilience. 'The Lord is my strength and my shield; my heart trusts in him, and he helps me' (Psalm 28:7).

9. Dear Lord, I pray against fear and worry that can weaken my faith and rob me of joy during this special time. Fill me with courage, trust, and confidence in Your unfailing love and plans for me and my baby. 'For God gave us a spirit not of fear but of power and love and self-control' (2 Timothy 1:7).

10. Loving Father, I thank You for Your promise of strength and protection in times of weakness and vulnerability. I place my trust in You and rely on Your grace to carry me through this pregnancy journey. 'The Lord is my strength and my song; he has become my salvation' (Psalm 118:14).

DAY 19: PRAYERS FOR A SUPER-NATURAL AND MIRACULOUS DELIVERY

1. Heavenly Father, I come before You with faith and expectation, believing in Your power to perform miracles. I pray for a supernatural and miraculous delivery of my baby, surpassing all natural limitations. 'Is anything too hard for the Lord?' (Genesis 18:14).

2. Lord, I surrender my delivery into Your hands, knowing that You are the author of life and the One who brings forth new beginnings. I invite Your divine presence to overshadow me, transforming the delivery into a supernatural encounter with Your glory. 'The Lord is near to all who call on him' (Psalm 145:18).

3. Gracious God, I pray for the supernatural alignment and positioning of my baby for optimal and smooth delivery. Guide their movements and rotations, ensuring they are in the perfect position for a safe and efficient birth. 'Commit your way to the Lord; trust in him, and he will act' (Psalm 37:5).

4. Dear Lord, I ask for supernatural pain relief and comfort during labor. Let Your divine presence bring peace and calmness, soothing any discomfort or intensity. Grant me a supernatural ability to endure and overcome the challenges of childbirth. 'I can do all things through him who strengthens me' (Philippians 4:13).

5. Loving Father, I pray for a supernatural acceleration of

the birthing process. May the stages of labor progress swiftly and smoothly, surpassing all natural expectations. I trust in Your perfect timing and divine intervention. 'But with God, all things are possible' (Matthew 19:26).

6. Heavenly Father, I pray for supernatural protection over me and my baby during the delivery. Shield us from any complications or risks, and let Your angels surround us, ensuring a safe and secure birth. 'The angel of the Lord encamps around those who fear him, and delivers them' (Psalm 34:7).

7. Lord, I pray for supernatural wisdom and discernment for my healthcare providers. May they be divinely guided in every decision, intervention, and action, ensuring the best possible outcome for me and my baby. 'If any of you lacks wisdom, let him ask God, who gives generously to all without reproach, and it will be given him' (James 1:5).

8. Gracious God, I ask for a supernatural release of joy and celebration in the delivery room. May the atmosphere be filled with Your presence, love, and peace, bringing a sense of awe and wonder as new life enters the world. 'You have turned for me my mourning into dancing; you have loosed my sackcloth and clothed me with gladness' (Psalm 30:11).

9. Dear Lord, I pray for a supernatural bonding and connection between me and my baby during and after delivery. Let our hearts intertwine, and may our love and attachment be deep and strong from the very first moments. 'And the two shall become one flesh' (Genesis 2:24).

10.   Loving Father, I thank You for the supernatural and extraordinary ways You work in our lives. I surrender my delivery to Your supernatural power and trust that You will exceed my expectations, bringing forth a miracle in the birth of my baby. 'Now to him who is able to do far more abundantly than all that we ask or think, according to the power at work within us' (Ephesians 3:20).

DAY 20: PRAYERS FOR COURAGE AND BOLDNESS

1. Heavenly Father, I pray for an infusion of courage and boldness as I journey through pregnancy. Help me to face each challenge with strength and resilience, knowing that You are with me. 'Be strong and courageous. Do not be afraid; do not be discouraged, for the Lord your God will be with you wherever you go' (Joshua 1:9).

2. Lord, I ask for the courage to embrace the changes and uncertainties that come with pregnancy. Grant me the boldness to step out of my comfort zone and trust in Your plans for me and my baby. 'For God has not given us a spirit of fear, but of power and of love and of a sound mind' (2 Timothy 1:7).

3. Gracious God, I pray for boldness to make decisions that align with Your will for me and my child. Give me the confidence to stand firm in my convictions and to seek Your guidance in all matters. 'The fear of man lays a snare, but whoever trusts in the Lord is safe' (Proverbs 29:25).

4. Dear Lord, I ask for courage and boldness to advocate for myself and my baby's well-being. Grant me the strength to speak up, ask questions, and assert my needs throughout this pregnancy journey. 'Have I not commanded you? Be strong and courageous. Do not be frightened, and do not be dismayed, for the Lord your God is with you wherever you go' (Joshua 1:9).

5. Loving Father, I pray for boldness to embrace the changes happening within my body with acceptance and grace. Help me to appreciate the beauty of pregnancy and to view it as a testament to Your amazing design. 'I praise you because I am fearfully and wonderfully made; your works are wonderful, I know that full well' (Psalm 139:14).

6. Heavenly Father, I ask for courage and boldness to overcome any fears or anxieties that may arise during pregnancy. Fill me with Your peace that surpasses all understanding and embolden me to trust in Your perfect plan for me and my baby. 'For God gave us a spirit not of fear but of power and love and self-control' (2 Timothy 1:7).

7. Lord, I pray for boldness to prioritize self-care and seek support when needed. Help me to recognize my limitations and to ask for help without hesitation or guilt. 'So do not fear, for I am with you; do not be dismayed, for I am your God. I will strengthen you and help you; I will uphold you with my righteous right hand' (Isaiah 41:10).

8. Gracious God, I ask for courage and boldness to embrace the challenges of motherhood that lie ahead. Grant me the confidence to trust in Your guidance and the ability to navigate the joys and difficulties with grace and perseverance. 'I can do all things through him who strengthens me' (Philippians 4:13).

9. Dear Lord, I pray for boldness to celebrate and share the joy of my pregnancy with others. Help me to radiate positivity, gratitude, and excitement, inspiring those around me with hope and encouragement. 'Let us hold

fast the confession of our hope without wavering, for he who promised is faithful' (Hebrews 10:23).

10.   Loving Father, I thank You for the gift of courage and boldness that You provide. Strengthen me in moments of weakness, embolden me to face challenges head-on, and help me to embrace the journey of pregnancy with unwavering faith. 'For God has not given us a spirit of fear, but of power and of love and of a sound mind' (2 Timothy 1:7).

DAY 21: PRAYERS FOR PROTECTION AGAINST EVIL ATTACKS DURING PREGNANCY

1. Heavenly Father, I come before You seeking Your divine protection against any evil attacks that may target me and my unborn child during this pregnancy. Surround us with Your heavenly angels and shield us from all forms of harm. 'The Lord will keep you from all evil; he will keep your life' (Psalm 121:7).

2. Lord, I pray for a hedge of spiritual protection around me and my baby. Guard us from any negative influences, spiritual attacks, or demonic forces that may seek to harm us. 'But the Lord is faithful. He will establish you and guard you against the evil one' (2 Thessalonians 3:3).

3. Gracious God, I ask for Your strength and power to resist any temptations or schemes of the enemy that may try to distract or lead me astray during this pregnancy. Grant me discernment to recognize and reject evil influences. 'Submit yourselves, then, to God. Resist the devil, and he will flee from you' (James 4:7).

4. Dear Lord, I pray for the protection of my mind, heart, and spirit against fear, anxiety, and negative thoughts. Fill me with Your peace and assurance, guarding me from any spiritual attacks that aim to rob me of joy and faith. 'For God gave us a spirit not of fear but of power and love and self-control' (2 Timothy 1:7).

5. Loving Father, I ask for Your divine covering over my dreams and sleep during this pregnancy. Protect me from nightmares, disturbing thoughts, or any form of spiritual attack that may disrupt my rest. 'In peace, I will both lie down and sleep; for you alone, O Lord, make me dwell in safety' (Psalm 4:8).

6. Heavenly Father, I pray for Your wisdom and guidance to discern and avoid any harmful influences or practices that may open doors to evil attacks. Help me to make choices that align with Your will and protect me from any spiritual vulnerabilities. 'I will instruct you and teach you in the way you should go; I will counsel you with my eye upon you' (Psalm 32:8).

7. Lord, I ask for Your grace and strength to resist any negative energy or words that may be spoken over me during this pregnancy. Shield me from harmful gossip, curses, or any form of verbal attack. 'No weapon that is fashioned against you shall succeed' (Isaiah 54:17).

8. Gracious God, I pray for the protection of my emotions and mental well-being during pregnancy. Guard me against excessive worry, stress, and mood fluctuations that may make me vulnerable to spiritual attacks. Fill me with Your peace and stability. 'The Lord is my rock and my fortress and my deliverer, my God, my rock, in whom I take refuge' (Psalm 18:2).

9. Dear Lord, I ask for Your divine intervention and protection against any physical ailments or complications that may arise as a result of evil attacks. Strengthen my body, immune system, and overall health, keeping me and my baby safe. 'He will cover you with his pinions,

and under his wings, you will find refuge; his faithfulness is a shield and buckler' (Psalm 91:4).

10.   Loving Father, I thank You for Your constant presence and protection. I trust in Your unfailing love and power to shield me and my baby from any evil attacks. I rest in the assurance that You are greater than any forces that may come against us. 'The Lord is my light and my salvation; whom shall I fear? The Lord is the stronghold of my life; of whom shall I be afraid?' (Psalm 27:1)."

DAY 22: PRAYERS FOR PROTECTION AGAINST DEATH FOR BOTH CHILD AND MOTHER

1. Heavenly Father, I come before You with a humble heart, seeking Your divine protection against the threat of death for both me and my unborn child. Guard us with Your loving presence and surround us with Your angels of protection. 'The Lord is my strength and my shield; my heart trusts in him, and he helps me' (Psalm 28:7).

2. Lord, I pray for a covering of Your life-giving power over me and my baby. Preserve our lives and shield us from any harm or danger that may lead to death. May Your hand of protection be upon us throughout this pregnancy journey. 'You are my hiding place; you will protect me from trouble and surround me with songs of deliverance' (Psalm 32:7).

3. Gracious God, I declare Your promise of abundant life over me and my child. I rebuke any spirit of death or destruction that may attempt to come against us. Fill us with Your divine vitality and protect us from premature death. 'The thief comes only to steal and kill and destroy; I have come that they may have life and have it to the full' (John 10:10).

4. Dear Lord, I pray for Your divine intervention to avert any health complications or unforeseen circumstances that may pose a risk to the lives of both me and my baby. Guide my healthcare providers and grant them wisdom in ensuring our well-being. 'Heal me, O Lord,

and I shall be healed; save me, and I shall be saved, for you are my praise' (Jeremiah 17:14).

5. Loving Father, I surrender our lives into Your loving hands, trusting in Your sovereign plan for us. Protect us from accidents, complications, or any other circumstances that could result in harm or death. Uphold us with Your righteous right hand. 'Fear not, for I am with you; be not dismayed, for I am your God; I will strengthen you, I will help you, I will uphold you with my righteous right hand' (Isaiah 41:10).

6. Heavenly Father, I pray for divine health and vitality to flow through every cell of our bodies. Strengthen our immune systems and protect us from any illnesses or diseases that could threaten our lives. Fill us with Your healing presence. 'Beloved, I pray that all may go well with you and that you may be in good health, as it goes well with your soul' (3 John 1:2).

7. Lord, I declare Your promises of long life and fulfillment of purpose over me and my child. Guard us against premature death and enable us to live out the plans and destinies You have ordained for us. 'For I know the plans I have for you,' declares the Lord, 'plans to prosper you and not to harm you, plans to give you hope and a future' (Jeremiah 29:11).

8. Gracious God, I pray for Your supernatural protection during childbirth. Safeguard both me and my baby from any complications or dangers that may arise during the delivery process. Grant us a safe and successful delivery. 'But you, Lord, are a shield around me, my glory, the One who lifts my head high' (Psalm 3:3).

9. Dear Lord, I lift up prayers of gratitude for the gift of life and the opportunity to bring forth a child into this world. Thank You for Your constant presence and protection. I trust in Your faithfulness to safeguard us from death and to watch over us with unfailing love. 'The Lord is faithful to all his promises and loving toward all he has made' (Psalm 145:13).

10.   Loving Father, I surrender all my fears and anxieties about the possibility of death for me or my child into Your hands. Fill me with Your peace that surpasses all understanding, knowing that You are our ultimate pro-tector and sustainer. 'When I am afraid, I put my trust in you' (Psalm 56:3).

DAY 23: PRAYERS FOR GIVING BIRTH TO A PERFECT AND COMPLETE CHILD

1. Heavenly Father, I come before You with a heart full of hope and anticipation, seeking Your divine intervention for the birth of a perfect and complete child. I place my trust in Your ability to form and shape my baby according to Your perfect design. 'For you created my inmost being; you knit me together in my mother's womb' (Psalm 139:13).

2. Lord, I surrender the development and growth of my baby into Your loving hands. I pray for every organ, limb, and system to form perfectly and function as intended. May my child be fearfully and wonderfully made, a testimony to Your marvelous works. 'I praise you because I am fearfully and wonderfully made; your works are wonderful, I know that full well' (Psalm 139:14).

3. Gracious God, I pray for the protection of my baby's physical and genetic makeup. Guard against any abnormalities or conditions that may hinder their health and well-being. Grant me peace and assurance in knowing that You are the giver of life and the sustainer of every living being. 'Every good and perfect gift is from above, coming down from the Father of the heavenly lights' (James 1:17).

4. Dear Lord, I declare that my baby is formed in Your image and likeness. I speak life, health, and completeness into every cell, tissue, and bone. May my child be bless-

ed with a sound mind, a strong body, and a heart that beats with love and compassion. 'So God created mankind in his own image, in the image of God he created them' (Genesis 1:27).

5. Loving Father, I pray for the growth and development of my baby's brain and cognitive abilities. Grant them wisdom, intelligence, and a thirst for knowledge. May their mind be sharp, creative, and receptive to learning. 'For the Lord gives wisdom; from his mouth come knowledge and understanding' (Proverbs 2:6).

6. Heavenly Father, I pray for the formation and strength of my baby's bones and muscles. May they develop with perfect symmetry and function. Grant my child agility, coordination, and physical strength to navigate the world with ease. 'He gives strength to the weary and increases the power of the weak' (Isaiah 40:29).

7. Lord, I lift up prayers for the development and health of my baby's senses. May their eyes see clearly, their ears hear joyfully, their taste buds savor the goodness of life, their nose perceive the beauty of fragrances, and their touch experience love and comfort. 'I praise you because I am fearfully and wonderfully made' (Psalm 139:14).

8. Gracious God, I pray for the formation and function of my baby's vital organs, including the heart, lungs, liver, and kidneys. May they develop and operate perfectly, sustaining life and promoting good health. I thank You for the intricate workings of the human body, a testament to Your wisdom and design. 'I will give thanks to you, for I am fearfully and wonderfully made' (Psalm 139:14).

9. Dear Lord, I surrender any worries or fears I may have about the well-being of my child. I trust in Your divine plan and purpose for their life. I believe that You have already ordained their days and have a beautiful future in store for them. 'For I know the plans I have for you,' declares the Lord, 'plans to prosper you and not to harm you, plans to give you hope and a future' (Jeremiah 29:11).

10. Loving Father, I thank You for the privilege of carrying this precious life within me. I pray for a safe and smooth delivery, bringing forth a perfect and complete child into the world. May they be a living testimony to Your goodness and faithfulness. In Your name, I pray. Amen.

DAY 24: PRAYERS FOR A PAIN-FREE AND COMPLICATION-FREE DELIVERY

1. Heavenly Father, I come before You with a heart full of faith, seeking Your divine intervention for a pain-free and complication-free delivery. I surrender all my fears and anxieties into Your hands, trusting in Your ability to guide and protect me. 'Do not be anxious about anything, but in every situation, by prayer and petition, with thanksgiving, present your requests to God' (Philippians 4:6).

2. Lord, I pray for Your supernatural presence to be with me throughout the labor and delivery process. Grant me strength, endurance, and a calm spirit. May Your peace envelop me, soothing any pain or discomfort. 'The Lord gives strength to his people; the Lord blesses his people with peace' (Psalm 29:11).

3. Gracious God, I ask for Your divine touch upon my body, preparing it for a smooth and easy delivery. Remove any obstacles or complications that may hinder the birthing process. Fill me with Your grace and favor, allowing everything to align perfectly for the safe arrival of my baby. 'With man this is impossible, but with God all things are possible' (Matthew 19:26).

4. Dear Lord, I pray for the guidance and wisdom of the medical professionals who will be attending to me during labor and delivery. Grant them skill, knowledge, and discernment in providing the necessary care. May their ac-

tions be guided by Your hand, ensuring the well-being of both me and my baby. 'By wisdom, a house is built, and through understanding, it is established' (Proverbs 24:3).

5. Loving Father, I declare Your peace and order over my body. I rebuke any complications or disruptions that may arise during the delivery process. May my body work in perfect harmony with Your divine design, bringing forth my baby with ease. 'For God is not a God of disorder but of peace' (1 Corinthians 14:33).

6. Heavenly Father, I pray for the quick and efficient progression of labor. Let the timing and intensity of contractions align perfectly, allowing my body to open and prepare for delivery. I trust in Your divine timing and provision. 'For everything there is a season, and a time for every matter under heaven' (Ecclesiastes 3:1).

7. Lord, I surrender my pain and discomfort to You. I ask for Your supernatural comfort and relief during labor. Pour out Your healing touch upon me, alleviating any physical distress. May Your presence be my source of strength and encouragement. 'Come to me, all you who are weary and burdened, and I will give you rest' (Matthew 11:28).

8. Gracious God, I pray for the proper positioning of my baby for delivery. Guide them into the optimal position for a smooth passage through the birth canal. Remove any hindrances or complications that may arise from improper positioning. 'Trust in the Lord with all your heart and lean not on your own understanding' (Proverbs 3:5).

9. Dear Lord, I pray for a quick recovery and healing after
the delivery. Strengthen my body, mind, and spirit as I
transition into the postpartum phase. Grant me rest, rejuvenation, and a smooth adjustment to the joys and challenges of motherhood. 'He gives strength to the weary
and increases the power of the weak' (Isaiah 40:29).

10.   Loving Father, I thank You in advance for the pain-
free and complication-free delivery I am about to experience. I trust in Your loving care and provision, knowing
that You are with me every step of the way. May Your
peace and joy fill the delivery room as I bring forth new
life. In Jesus' name, I pray. Amen.

DAY 25: PRAYERS FOR LONG LIFE AND PROSPERITY FOR MOTHER AND UNBORN CHILD

1. Heavenly Father, I lift up prayers of gratitude for the gift of life and the opportunity to nurture and raise this precious child. I pray for Your divine favor and blessing of long life and prosperity for both me and my unborn child. 'The fear of the Lord adds length to life, but the years of the wicked are cut short' (Proverbs 10:27).

2. Lord, I declare Your promises of abundant life and prosperity over me and my baby. I trust in Your provision and guidance in every aspect of our lives. May we experience the fullness of Your blessings and walk in the path of prosperity You have set before us. 'The Lord will grant you abundant prosperity' (Deuteronomy 28:11).

3. Gracious God, I pray for physical health, vitality, and well-being for both me and my unborn child. Strengthen our bodies, boost our immune systems, and protect us from any diseases or illnesses that may hinder our long life and prosperity. 'Beloved, I pray that all may go well with you and that you may be in good health, as it goes well with your soul' (3 John 1:2).

4. Dear Lord, I surrender all worries and anxieties about our financial well-being into Your hands. I trust in Your provision and abundance. May You open doors of opportunity, bless the work of our hands, and guide us in making wise financial decisions. 'The Lord will send a blessing on your barns and on everything you put your

hand to' (Deuteronomy 28:8).

5. Loving Father, I pray for a spirit of wisdom and discernment to be upon me as I make decisions that impact our lives. Grant me the insight to prioritize what truly matters, to make choices that align with Your will, and to cultivate a legacy of long life and prosperity for my child. 'For the Lord gives wisdom; from his mouth come knowledge and understanding' (Proverbs 2:6).

6. Heavenly Father, I declare Your promises of protection over our lives. Guard us from accidents, harm, and any dangers that may threaten our well-being. Surround us with Your angels of protection and keep us safe under Your loving care. 'He will command his angels concerning you to guard you in all your ways' (Psalm 91:11).

7. Lord, I pray for a spirit of generosity and abundance to flow through our lives. May we be blessed to bless others, to sow seeds of kindness, and to contribute to the well-being of those in need. Let our lives be a testimony of Your goodness and grace. 'Remember this: Whoever sows sparingly will also reap sparingly, and whoever sows generously will also reap generously' (2 Corinthians 9:6).

8. Gracious God, I pray for a strong and nurturing community around us, filled with supportive relationships and opportunities for growth. Surround us with positive influences, mentors, and friends who will contribute to our long life and prosperity. 'Two are better than one, because they have a good return for their labor' (Ecclesiastes 4:9).

9. Dear Lord, I surrender all worries and fears about the future into Your hands. I trust in Your divine plan for our lives, knowing that You have good things in store for us. Grant us the faith to step into the abundance and long life You have ordained for us. 'For I know the plans I have for you,' declares the Lord, 'plans to prosper you and not to harm you, plans to give you hope and a future' (Jeremiah 29:11).

10.   Loving Father, I thank You for Your faithfulness and Your promises of long life and prosperity. I place my trust in You, knowing that You are the source of all blessings. May our lives be filled with joy, abundance, and the testimony of Your goodness. In Jesus' name, I pray. Amen.

DAY 26: PRAYER FOR HUSBAND AND WIFE DURING THE PREGNANCY JOURNEY

1. Heavenly Father, I come before You with a heart full of gratitude for the blessing of pregnancy. I lift up my husband and myself as we embark on this journey together. May our love, support, and unity grow stronger as we prepare to welcome our child into the world. 'Two are better than one because they have a good return for their labor' (Ecclesiastes 4:9).

2. Lord, I pray for my husband's strength and wisdom as he supports me during this pregnancy. Grant him patience, understanding, and empathy to navigate the changes and challenges we may face. May his love and care be a reflection of Your unwavering love for us. 'Husbands, love your wives, just as Christ loved the church' (Ephesians 5:25).

3. Gracious God, bless our relationship with open communication and vulnerability. Help us to share our fears, hopes, and dreams with one another. May our conversations be filled with grace, understanding, and encouragement, fostering a deeper connection as we journey through this precious season. 'Therefore encourage one another and build one another up' (1 Thessalonians 5:11).

4. Dear Lord, I pray for a spirit of unity and teamwork between my husband and me. May we approach the challenges and decisions of pregnancy with a shared vision

and a united front. Guide us in making choices that honor You and prioritize the well-being of our family. 'Make every effort to keep the unity of the Spirit through the bond of peace' (Ephesians 4:3).

5. Loving Father, I pray for emotional support and stability for both my husband and me. Shield us from anxiety, stress, and hormonal fluctuations that may affect our emotions. Fill our hearts with Your peace, joy, and gratitude as we embrace this miraculous journey together. 'Cast all your anxiety on him because he cares for you' (1 Peter 5:7).

6. Heavenly Father, I pray for my husband's role as a provider for our growing family. Grant him the wisdom, strength, and favor in his work or business endeavors. May he find fulfillment and joy in his responsibilities, knowing that You are the ultimate provider for our needs. 'And my God will meet all your needs according to the riches of his glory in Christ Jesus' (Philippians 4:19).

7. Lord, I lift up prayers for our spiritual growth and alignment as a couple. May we seek You together, studying Your Word, praying, and worshiping as a united front. Strengthen our faith individually and as a family, guiding us in raising our child in the ways of Your truth and love. 'But as for me and my household, we will serve the Lord' (Joshua 24:15).

8. Gracious God, I pray for physical and emotional well-being for both my husband and me during this pregnancy. Protect us from any illnesses, complications, or discomforts that may arise. Grant us the energy, vitality, and rest we need to navigate this journey with grace. 'The

Lord is my strength and my shield; my heart trusts in him, and he helps me' (Psalm 28:7).

9. Dear Lord, I pray for moments of joy, laughter, and bonding between my husband and me as we anticipate the arrival of our child. May we create cherished memories, enjoy quality time together, and build a strong foundation of love and affection. 'A time to weep and a time to laugh, a time to mourn and a time to dance' (Ecclesiastes 3:4).

10. Loving Father, I thank You for the gift of my husband and the strength of our partnership. I commit our relationship, our pregnancy, and our future as parents into Your loving hands. May You continue to bless and guide us every step of the way. In Jesus' name, I pray. Amen.

DAY 27: PRAYER FOR PATIENCE AND GRACE DURING THE PREGNANCY JOURNEY

1. Heavenly Father, I come before You with a humble heart, seeking Your grace and patience as my husband and I journey through the ups and downs of pregnancy. Grant us the ability to extend patience and understanding to one another, embracing the changes and challenges with grace. 'Be completely humble and gentle; be patient, bearing with one another in love' (Ephesians 4:2).

2. Lord, I pray for patience in times of physical discomfort and fatigue. Help us to remain calm and composed, knowing that this temporary phase is part of the miraculous process of bringing new life into the world. Grant us the strength to endure with patience and trust in Your perfect timing. 'But if we hope for what we do not yet have, we wait for it patiently' (Romans 8:25).

3. Gracious God, I pray for patience in navigating the emotional highs and lows that pregnancy brings. Fill our hearts with compassion and understanding, allowing us to offer grace to one another when emotions are heightened. Help us to communicate with love and kindness, seeking to bring comfort and support. 'Love is patient, love is kind' (1 Corinthians 13:4).

4. Dear Lord, I pray for patience in making decisions and preparations for the arrival of our baby. Guide us in choosing the right healthcare providers, making informed choices about birthing plans, and creating a nur-

turing environment for our child. Grant us discernment and patience as we navigate through the multitude of options before us. 'Commit to the Lord whatever you do, and he will establish your plans' (Proverbs 16:3).

5. Loving Father, I pray for patience in waiting for the milestones and developments of pregnancy. Help us to trust in Your perfect timing and to find joy in each stage of our baby's growth. May we embrace the journey with a patient and grateful heart, knowing that Your plans for our child are unfolding beautifully. 'The Lord is good to those who wait for him' (Lamentations 3:25).

6. Heavenly Father, I pray for patience in accepting our limitations and seeking help when needed. Teach us to rely on You and lean on our support system during times of physical and emotional strain. Help us to release any feelings of guilt or inadequacy, understanding that asking for help is a sign of strength. 'For when I am weak, then I am strong' (2 Corinthians 12:10).

7. Lord, I lift up prayers for patience in our interactions with others during this pregnancy journey. Grant us the ability to handle unsolicited advice or opinions with grace and humility. Help us to focus on what is best for our family and to respond with patience and love. 'A gentle answer turns away wrath, but a harsh word stirs up anger' (Proverbs 15:1).

8. Gracious God, I pray for patience in the face of unexpected challenges or complications that may arise during pregnancy. Fill us with faith and trust in Your sovereignty, knowing that You are in control and working all things together for our good. Give us the patience to endure

and the hope to persevere. 'And endurance produces character, and character produces hope' (Romans 5:4).

9. Dear Lord, I pray for patience in our relationship with You. Help us to surrender our worries, fears, and uncertainties into Your hands, trusting that You will provide and guide us through this journey. Teach us to find peace and rest in Your presence, knowing that You are working for our good. 'Wait for the Lord; be strong, and let your heart take courage; wait for the Lord!' (Psalm 27:14).

10.   Loving Father, I thank You for Your endless patience and grace toward us. As we navigate the pregnancy journey, I pray that Your patience and grace would overflow within us, enabling us to love one another deeply and unconditionally. In Jesus' name, I pray. Amen.

DAY 28: PRAYER FOR A CLOSER WALK WITH GOD DURING AND AFTER PREGNANCY

1. Heavenly Father, I come before You with a desire for a closer walk with You during and after this pregnancy. Draw me near to Your presence, that I may experience Your love, guidance, and comfort in a deeper way. 'Draw near to God, and he will draw near to you' (James 4:8).

2. Lord, I pray for a hunger and thirst for Your Word. May the Scriptures come alive to me, providing wisdom, strength, and encouragement for this season of pregnancy and motherhood. Help me to prioritize time in Your Word and allow it to shape my thoughts and actions. 'Your word is a lamp to my feet and a light to my path' (Psalm 119:105).

3. Gracious God, I pray for a consistent and fervent prayer life. Teach me to seek Your face and pour out my heart before You in all circumstances. May prayer become a source of comfort, peace, and intimate connection with You. 'Pray without ceasing' (1 Thessalonians 5:17).

4. Dear Lord, I pray for a surrendered heart. Help me to surrender my plans, fears, and desires to You, trusting in Your perfect will for my life and the life of my child. May I find peace in knowing that You are in control and that Your plans are higher than my own. 'Commit your way to the Lord; trust in him, and he will act' (Psalm 37:5).

5. Loving Father, I pray for a spirit of gratitude and praise. Open my eyes to the countless blessings around me, even in the midst of pregnancy challenges. Help me to cultivate a heart of thanksgiving, acknowledging Your goodness and faithfulness in every season. 'Give thanks in all circumstances; for this is the will of God in Christ Jesus for you' (1 Thessalonians 5:18).

6. Heavenly Father, I pray for fellowship with other believers. Surround me with a supportive community of faith that will encourage, uplift, and sharpen me in my walk with You. May we spur one another on toward love and good deeds, sharing the journey of motherhood and faith together. 'And let us consider how to stir up one another to love and good works, not neglecting to meet together, as is the habit of some, but encouraging one another' (Hebrews 10:24-25).

7. Lord, I pray for a discerning spirit. Grant me wisdom and discernment as I make decisions regarding my own spiritual growth, as well as the influences and teachings that will shape my child's faith. Help me to choose wisely, aligning myself with those who will lead me closer to You. 'The fear of the Lord is the beginning of wisdom, and the knowledge of the Holy One is insight' (Proverbs 9:10).

8. Gracious God, I pray for a heart of worship. Fill my soul with awe and reverence for You, even in the midst of the busyness and demands of pregnancy and motherhood. Help me to worship You in spirit and in truth, offering my life as a living sacrifice to honor and glorify You. 'Yet a time is coming and has now come when the true wor-

shipers will worship the Father in the Spirit and in truth, for they are the kind of worshipers the Father seeks' (John 4:23).

9. Dear Lord, I pray for a renewed passion for serving others. Open my eyes to the needs of those around me, both within and outside of my family. Guide me in using my gifts, time, and resources to bless others and be a reflection of Your love and compassion. 'For even the Son of Man came not to be served but to serve, and to give his life as a ransom for many' (Mark 10:45).

10.   Loving Father, I commit myself and my child into Your hands. May our journey through pregnancy and motherhood deepen my relationship with You, as I trust in Your unfailing love and faithfulness. Help me to walk closely with You, seeking Your will and following Your guidance all the days of my life. In Jesus' name, I pray. Amen.

DAY 29: PRAYER FOR A HEALTHY AND STRESS-FREE PREGNANCY

1. Heavenly Father, I come before You with a heart full of gratitude for the gift of pregnancy. I pray for an inch-free pregnancy period, free from complications, sickness, and stress. Cover me and my unborn child with Your protective and healing hand. 'Surely he will save you from the fowler's snare and from the deadly pestilence' (Psalm 91:3).

2. Lord, I pray for the health and well-being of my body during this pregnancy. Strengthen my immune system, protect me from infections, and keep me in optimal health. Grant me the energy and vitality I need to carry this child with ease. 'Beloved, I pray that all may go well with you and that you may be in good health, as it goes well with your soul' (3 John 1:2).

3. Gracious God, I pray against any complications or abnormalities that could arise during this pregnancy. I ask for Your divine intervention and protection, that every aspect of the development of my baby would be perfect and in accordance with Your design. 'For you formed my inward parts; you knitted me together in my mother's womb' (Psalm 139:13).

4. Dear Lord, I surrender all my fears and anxieties about the well-being of my baby into Your hands. Replace my worries with Your peace that surpasses all understanding. Help me to trust in Your divine plan and to rest in the knowledge that You are in control. 'Do not be anxious

about anything, but in every situation, by prayer and petition, with thanksgiving, present your requests to God'
(Philippians 4:6).

5. Loving Father, I pray for a stress-free pregnancy. Help
   me to manage any stressors or anxieties that may arise
   during this time. Grant me the ability to find peace and
   tranquility in Your presence, and to cast all my cares
   upon You. 'Come to me, all who labor and are heavy
   laden, and I will give you rest' (Matthew 11:28).

6. Heavenly Father, I pray for a healthy and balanced lifestyle during this pregnancy. Guide me in making wise
   choices regarding nutrition, exercise, rest, and self-care.
   Help me to prioritize my well-being and the well-being
   of my baby, following Your leading in every aspect. 'Or
   do you not know that your body is a temple of the Holy
   Spirit within you, whom you have from God? You are not
   your own' (1 Corinthians 6:19).

7. Lord, I pray for protection from any external factors that
   may pose a threat to the health of my baby and myself.
   Shield us from harm, accidents, and any form of danger.
   Surround us with Your divine protection and keep us safe
   under Your wings. 'He will cover you with his feathers,
   and under his wings you will find refuge; his faithfulness
   will be your shield and rampart' (Psalm 91:4).

8. Gracious God, I pray for a supportive and understanding
   network of family, friends, and healthcare providers who
   will journey with me through this pregnancy. Surround
   me with individuals who will uplift, encourage, and provide the necessary care and guidance. 'Two are better
   than one, because they have a good reward for their toil'

(Ecclesiastes 4:9).

9. Dear Lord, I commit my pregnancy into Your hands, trusting that You have plans for my child's life and mine. Give me the assurance that You are watching over us, guiding us, and working all things for our good. Help me to surrender any fears or doubts and to embrace the joy and blessings of this pregnancy. 'For I know the plans I have for you,' declares the Lord, 'plans to prosper you and not to harm you, plans to give you hope and a future' (Jeremiah 29:11).

10. Loving Father, I thank You in advance for a healthy and inch-free pregnancy period. I place my faith and confidence in Your unfailing love and faithfulness. May this pregnancy be a testimony of Your miraculous power and grace. In Jesus' name, I pray. Amen.

DAY 30: PRAYER FOR GRACE AND STRENGTH DURING PREGNANCY

1. Heavenly Father, I come before You with a humble heart, seeking Your grace and strength for my husband and myself as we journey through this pregnancy. Pour out Your abundant grace upon us, empowering us to face the challenges and joys that lie ahead. 'But he said to me, "My grace is sufficient for you, for my power is made perfect in weakness."' (2 Corinthians 12:9).

2. Lord, I pray for emotional strength and stability for both my husband and myself. Pregnancy can bring about a range of emotions, from excitement and happiness to worry and anxiety. Fill our hearts with Your peace, comfort, and stability, enabling us to navigate these emotions with grace. 'Do not be anxious about anything, but in every situation, by prayer and petition, with thanksgiving, present your requests to God' (Philippians 4:6).

3. Gracious God, I pray for physical strength and vitality for both of us. Pregnancy can be physically demanding, but I know that You are our strength and sustainer. Grant us the energy and endurance we need to carry on with our daily tasks and responsibilities. 'I can do all things through him who strengthens me' (Philippians 4:13).

4. Dear Lord, I pray for mental clarity and wisdom. Help us to make informed decisions regarding our health, well-being, and the well-being of our unborn child. Guide us in seeking appropriate medical care, adopting healthy habits, and making choices that align with Your

will. 'If any of you lacks wisdom, let him ask God, who gives generously to all without reproach, and it will be given him' (James 1:5).

5. Loving Father, I pray for spiritual strength and growth during this pregnancy. May this season draw us closer to You and deepen our faith in Your unfailing love and provision. Help us to rely on Your wisdom and guidance, seeking Your will in all areas of our lives. 'Trust in the Lord with all your heart, and do not lean on your own understanding' (Proverbs 3:5).

6. Heavenly Father, I pray for unity and harmony in our marriage as we embark on this journey of parenthood. Strengthen the bond between us, deepening our love, respect, and communication. Help us to support and encourage one another, sharing the responsibilities and joys of pregnancy together. 'Two are better than one, because they have a good reward for their toil' (Ecclesiastes 4:9).

7. Lord, I pray for patience and grace during moments of discomfort and uncertainty. Pregnancy can bring about physical and emotional challenges, but I trust that You will sustain us. Help us to lean on Your grace and to exhibit patience and understanding towards one another. 'With all humility and gentleness, with patience, bearing with one another in love' (Ephesians 4:2).

8. Gracious God, I pray for wisdom in nurturing a healthy and loving environment for our unborn child. Guide us in making choices that will create a positive atmosphere filled with love, peace, and joy. May our home be a place where our child feels safe, cherished, and encouraged.

'Train up a child in the way he should go; even when he is old he will not depart from it' (Proverbs 22:6).

9. Dear Lord, I surrender my fears and anxieties about the future into Your hands. Help us to trust in Your perfect timing and provision. Fill us with confidence and hope, knowing that You are with us every step of the way. 'For I know the plans I have for you,' declares the Lord, 'plans to prosper you and not to harm you, plans to give you hope and a future' (Jeremiah 29:11).

10. Loving Father, I thank You for Your grace and strength that sustains us. As we walk this journey of pregnancy together, may Your presence be evident in our lives. Grant us the wisdom, patience, and love we need to embrace this season wholeheartedly. In Jesus' name, I pray. Amen.

DAY 31: PRAYER OF THANKSGIVING AND FAITH FOR A SUCCESSFUL PREGNANCY

1. Heavenly Father, I come before You with a heart filled with gratitude for the blessing of pregnancy. Thank You for entrusting me with the gift of carrying life within me. I offer my heartfelt thanksgiving for this miracle and the joy it brings. 'Give thanks to the Lord, for he is good; his love endures forever' (Psalm 107:1).

2. Lord, I thank You for the strength and endurance You have given me throughout this pregnancy journey. Thank You for sustaining me through the ups and downs, the challenges and triumphs. I am grateful for Your faithfulness and for the assurance that You will continue to uphold me. 'The Lord is my strength and my shield; my heart trusts in him, and he helps me' (Psalm 28:7).

3. Gracious God, I express my gratitude for the health and well-being of both me and my unborn child. Thank You for the precious life growing within me and for the protection You have provided. I am grateful for the milestones reached, the healthy development, and the signs of vitality. 'I will give thanks to you, Lord, with all my heart; I will tell of all your wonderful deeds' (Psalm 9:1).

4. Dear Lord, I thank You for the wisdom and guidance You have bestowed upon me during this pregnancy. Thank You for the discernment to make informed decisions, for leading me to the right healthcare providers, and for surrounding me with a supportive network. I am grateful

for Your provision and guidance every step of the way. 'Trust in the Lord with all your heart and lean not on your own understanding' (Proverbs 3:5).

5. Loving Father, I offer my thanks for the moments of joy and anticipation that pregnancy brings. Thank You for the first flutters and kicks, for the shared excitement with loved ones, and for the dreams and hopes that have taken root in my heart. I am grateful for the privilege of experiencing this miracle of life. 'You have turned my mourning into joyful dancing. You have taken away my clothes of mourning and clothed me with joy' (Psalm 30:11).

6. Heavenly Father, I express my gratitude for the bond that is forming between me and my unborn child. Thank You for the precious moments of connection, for the love that grows with each passing day. I am grateful for the privilege of nurturing and caring for this little one. 'For you created my inmost being; you knit me together in my mother's womb' (Psalm 139:13).

7. Lord, I thank You for the lessons of patience and surrender that pregnancy teaches. Thank You for reminding me of the beauty of Your timing and for teaching me to trust in Your plans. I am grateful for the opportunity to grow in faith and reliance on You. 'Be still before the Lord and wait patiently for him; do not fret when people succeed in their ways' (Psalm 37:7).

8. Gracious God, I thank You for the support and love of my spouse, family, and friends. Thank You for their encouragement, prayers, and presence throughout this pregnancy. I am grateful for the community that surrounds

me, lifting me up and sharing in the excitement of this journey. 'Two are better than one because they have a good return for their labor' (Ecclesiastes 4:9).

9. Dear Lord, I offer my gratitude for the moments of peace and serenity amidst the busyness of pregnancy. Thank You for the times of quiet reflection, for the assurance of Your presence, and for the reassurance that You are in control. I am grateful for the moments of stillness that bring me closer to You. 'Be still, and know that I am God' (Psalm 46:10).

10.	Loving Father, I express my faith and trust in You for a successful pregnancy and a safe delivery. I believe that You are faithful to complete the work You have begun in me. I place my confidence in Your loving care and provision, knowing that You will bring forth new life according to Your perfect plan. 'Now faith is confidence in what we hope for and assurance about what we do not see' (Hebrews 11:1). In Jesus' name, I offer this prayer of thanksgiving and faith. Amen.

POST-PARTUM PERIOD

The post-partum period is a time of healing, recovery, and adjustment for new mothers. It is a season that brings with it unique challenges and emotions. In this collection of post-partum prayers, we invite you to journey through seven days of intentional prayer and reflection, seeking God's comfort, healing, and guidance.

Each day's prayers are designed to address specific aspects of post-partum recovery, including physical healing, emotional well-being, protection against post-partum depression, and the need for faith, thanksgiving, and help. These prayers are accompanied by selected Bible verses, offering inspiration, strength, and reassurance as you navigate this tender season.

Through these prayers, I encourage you to surrender your worries, fears, and burdens to God, trusting in His love, provision, and guidance. We invite you to cultivate an attitude of gratitude, recognizing the blessings and joys that come with motherhood. May these prayers serve as a reminder that you are not alone on this journey and that God is with you every step of the way.

Whether you are a new mother or have experienced post-partum before, these prayers are meant to provide solace, encouragement, and a sense of connection to the Divine. Take a few moments each day to quiet your heart, seek God's presence, and pour out your concerns, hopes, and praises. May these prayers bring you comfort, strength, and a deepening faith as you embrace the miraculous gift of motherhood and navigate the beautiful complexities of the post-partum period.

The prayers are designed to be prayed every day for 7 days, that this the whole week and you should repeat the prayer circle. God bless you super mum, you have done a great job. You have done well.

MONDAYS POST-PARTUM PRAYERS

1. Heavenly Father, I thank You for the safe delivery of my baby. I pray for complete healing and restoration for my body. Grant me strength and energy as I recover. "He heals the brokenhearted and binds up their wounds." - Psalm 147:3

2. Lord, I lift up my emotions to You. Help me navigate the changes and challenges that come with being a new mother. Grant me patience, peace, and joy in this season. "May the God of hope fill you with all joy and peace in believing, so that by the power of the Holy Spirit you may abound in hope." - Romans 15:13

3. Gracious God, I pray for wisdom and guidance as I care for my newborn. Help me to understand their needs and respond with love and patience. Surround me with supportive individuals who can offer guidance and assistance. "If any of you lacks wisdom, let him ask God, who gives generously to all without reproach, and it will be given him." - James 1:5

4. Lord, I surrender my fears and anxieties about motherhood to You. Fill me with confidence and assurance that You have equipped me for this journey. Help me to trust in Your provision and rely on Your strength. "I can do all things through him who strengthens me." - Philippians 4:13

5. Heavenly Father, I pray for the bonding between me and my baby. Let our love and connection grow stron-

ger each day. Grant me patience and understanding as we navigate this new relationship. "Love is patient and kind... Love bears all things, believes all things, hopes all things, endures all things." - 1 Corinthians 13:4,7

6. Lord, I lift up any sleep deprivation or exhaustion I may be experiencing. Grant me peaceful and restful sleep when I have the opportunity to rest. Strengthen me physically and mentally to handle the demands of motherhood. "It is in vain that you rise up early and go late to rest, eating the bread of anxious toil; for he gives to his beloved sleep." - Psalm 127:2

7. Gracious God, I pray for emotional well-being and mental health during this post-partum period. Guard my mind from negative thoughts and fill me with peace and joy. Surround me with understanding and supportive individuals who can offer encouragement and assistance. "For God gave us a spirit not of fear but of power and love and self-control." - 2 Timothy 1:7

TUESDAYS POST-PARTUM PRAYERS

1. Heavenly Father, I thank You for the gift of motherhood. Help me embrace this new role with grace and humility. Grant me wisdom and strength as I navigate the joys and challenges of raising my child. "Behold, children are a heritage from the Lord, the fruit of the womb a reward." - Psalm 127:3

2. Lord, I pray for patience and understanding as I adjust to the demands of caring for a newborn. Help me to be present in each moment and cherish the precious time I have with my baby. "So teach us to number our days that we may get a heart of wisdom." - Psalm 90:12

3. Gracious God, I surrender any feelings of inadequacy or self-doubt to You. Remind me that You have chosen me to be the mother of this child, and You will equip me with everything I need. Fill me with confidence and assurance in Your plan for my life. "I praise you, for I am fearfully and wonderfully made. Wonderful are your works; my soul knows it very well." - Psalm 139:14

4. Lord, I pray for strength and energy to meet the physical demands of motherhood. Renew my body and grant me good health. Help me to prioritize self-care and seek support when needed. "Do you not know that you are God's temple and that God's Spirit dwells in you? If anyone destroys God's temple, God will destroy him. For God's temple is holy, and you are that temple." - 1 Corinthians 3:16-17

5. Heavenly Father, I lift up my emotions to You. Guard my heart and mind from post-partum blues or depression. Surround me with understanding and supportive individuals who can offer comfort and encouragement. "The Lord is near to the brokenhearted and saves the crushed in spirit." - Psalm 34:18

6. Lord, I pray for wisdom and discernment as I make decisions regarding the care and upbringing of my child. Help me to seek Your guidance in all aspects of parenting. Grant me patience, understanding, and a heart filled with love. "Trust in the Lord with all your heart, and do not lean on your own understanding. In all your ways acknowledge him, and he will make straight your paths." - Proverbs 3:5-6

7. Gracious God, I lift up any feelings of guilt or self-criticism I may be experiencing as a new mother. Help me to let go of unrealistic expectations and embrace the journey of motherhood with grace and self-compassion. "For by grace you have been saved through faith. And this is not your own doing; it is the gift of God." - Ephesians 2:8

WEDNESDAYS POST-PARTUM PRAYERS:

1. Heavenly Father, I thank You for the precious gift of my child. Help me to cherish and nurture them with love and compassion. Grant me the wisdom to guide them on the path of righteousness. "Train up a child in the way he should go; even when he is old, he will not depart from it." - Proverbs 22:6

2. Lord, I pray for patience and grace as I navigate the challenges of breastfeeding. Grant me the ability to provide nourishment and comfort to my baby. Surround me with support and resources to help me succeed in this journey. "Like newborn infants, long for the pure spiritual milk, that by it you may grow up into salvation." - 1 Peter 2:2

3. Gracious God, I surrender any feelings of comparison or inadequacy to You. Help me to embrace my unique journey as a mother and not be swayed by societal expectations. Fill me with confidence in my abilities and remind me that You have chosen me for this role. "But he said to me, 'My grace is sufficient for you, for my power is made perfect in weakness.'" - 2 Corinthians 12:9

4. Lord, I pray for wisdom and discernment in setting boundaries and establishing routines for my baby. Help me to create a safe and nurturing environment that promotes their physical, emotional, and spiritual well-being. "For God is not a God of confusion but of peace." - 1

Corinthians 14:33

5. Heavenly Father, I lift up any feelings of exhaustion or overwhelm I may be experiencing. Grant me restful sleep and renewal of strength. Help me to prioritize self-care and seek support from my loved ones. "It is in vain that you rise up early and go late to rest, eating the bread of anxious toil; for he gives to his beloved sleep." - Psalm 127:2

6. Lord, I pray for the health and well-being of my baby. Protect them from illness and harm. Grant them strength, vitality, and a joyful spirit. "He will cover you with his pinions, and under his wings you will find refuge; his faithfulness is a shield and buckler." - Psalm 91:4

7. Gracious God, I surrender any fears or worries about my ability to be a good mother. Help me to trust in Your provision and seek Your guidance in every decision. Fill me with love, patience, and a nurturing spirit as I care for my child. "And these words that I command you today shall be on your heart. You shall teach them diligently to your children and shall talk of them when you sit in your house, and when you walk by the way, and when you lie down, and when you rise." - Deuteronomy 6:6-7

THURSDAYS POST-PARTUM PRAYERS

1. Heavenly Father, I thank You for Your faithfulness and for the healing that has taken place in my body since giving birth. I pray for a complete and speedy recovery. Grant me strength and resilience as I regain my physical well-being. "But he was pierced for our transgressions; he was crushed for our iniquities; upon him was the chastisement that brought us peace, and with his wounds, we are healed." - Isaiah 53:5

2. Lord, I lift up any discomfort or pain I may be experiencing. Bring relief and comfort to my body. I pray for the healing touch of Your hand upon me, restoring me to full health and vitality. "He heals the brokenhearted and binds up their wounds." - Psalm 147:3

3. Gracious God, I surrender any feelings of exhaustion or fatigue to You. Renew my strength and energy. Help me to find moments of rest and rejuvenation amidst the demands of caring for my baby. "Come to me, all who labor and are heavy laden, and I will give you rest." - Matthew 11:28

4. Lord, I pray for emotional healing and stability during this post-partum period. Guard my heart and mind from anxiety, stress, and overwhelm. Fill me with peace and joy as I embrace the joys and challenges of motherhood. "Cast all your anxieties on him because he cares for you." - 1 Peter 5:7

5. Heavenly Father, I surrender any feelings of self-doubt or guilt regarding my ability to care for my baby. Help me to be kind and gentle with myself, knowing that I am doing my best. Fill me with confidence and assurance in Your plan for me as a mother. "I praise you, for I am fearfully and wonderfully made. Wonderful are your works; my soul knows it very well." - Psalm 139:14

6. Lord, I pray for emotional and mental well-being during this post-partum period. Shield me from the baby blues or postpartum depression. Surround me with a supportive network of loved ones who can provide comfort, encouragement, and understanding. "The Lord is near to the brokenhearted and saves the crushed in spirit." - Psalm 34:18

7. Gracious God, I surrender any feelings of impatience or frustration as I navigate the challenges of recovery. Grant me grace and resilience as I embrace the healing process. Help me to be patient with my body and trust in Your perfect timing. "But they who wait for the Lord shall renew their strength; they shall mount up with wings like eagles; they shall run and not be weary; they shall walk and not faint." - Isaiah 40:31

FRIDAYS POST-PARTUM PRAYERS

1. Heavenly Father, I thank You for the miraculous journey of childbirth and the strength You have given me. I pray for continued healing and restoration of my body. May Your healing power flow through me, bringing complete healing to every part of me. "But I will restore you to health and heal your wounds," declares the Lord. - Jeremiah 30:17

2. Lord, I lift up any lingering physical discomfort or pain that I may be experiencing. I ask for Your touch to bring relief and restoration. Renew my body from the inside out, bringing healing to any areas that are still recovering. "He heals the brokenhearted and binds up their wounds." - Psalm 147:3

3. Gracious God, I surrender any feelings of fatigue or exhaustion to You. Strengthen me and renew my energy. Fill me with vitality and vigor as I care for my baby and attend to my own needs. "He gives strength to the weary and increases the power of the weak." - Isaiah 40:29

4. Lord, I pray for emotional healing and stability during this post-partum period. Guard my heart and mind from negative thoughts and emotions. Surround me with Your peace and fill me with Your joy. Help me to find comfort and solace in Your presence. "You will keep in perfect peace those whose minds are steadfast because they trust in you." - Isaiah 26:3

5. Heavenly Father, I surrender any feelings of overwhelm

or stress to You. Grant me a sense of calm and serenity as I adjust to the demands of motherhood. Help me to find balance and establish healthy routines. "Come to me, all you who are weary and burdened, and I will give you rest." - Matthew 11:28

6. Lord, I pray for the restoration of my emotional well-being. Heal any emotional wounds or traumas that may have surfaced during childbirth. Grant me inner strength and resilience. Surround me with loving and supportive relationships that nurture and uplift my spirit. "The Lord is close to the brokenhearted and saves those who are crushed in spirit." - Psalm 34:18

7. Gracious God, I surrender any feelings of self-doubt or inadequacy to You. Fill me with confidence and assurance in my abilities as a mother. Help me to embrace my unique journey and trust in Your wisdom and guidance. "I can do all this through him who gives me strength." - Philippians 4:13

SATURDAYS POST-PARTUM PRAYERS

1. Heavenly Father, I come before You and surrender any fears or anxieties I have about post-partum depression. I pray for Your protection over my mental and emotional well-being. Surround me with Your peace and joy, guarding my mind from negative thoughts and emotions. "For God has not given us a spirit of fear, but of power and of love and of a sound mind." - 2 Timothy 1:7

2. Lord, I pray for an outpouring of Your love and grace upon my heart. Fill me with Your perfect love that casts out all fear and brings healing to any emotional wounds. Help me to embrace my identity as a beloved child of God and to find solace in Your presence. "There is no fear in love. But perfect love drives out fear." - 1 John 4:18

3. Gracious God, I surrender any feelings of sadness or hopelessness to You. Renew my mind and fill me with Your peace that surpasses all understanding. Help me to focus on the blessings and joys of motherhood, finding gratitude in every moment. "The Lord is my strength and my shield; my heart trusts in him, and he helps me. My heart leaps for joy, and with my song I praise him." - Psalm 28:7

4. Lord, I pray for the support and understanding of my loved ones during this vulnerable time. Surround me with individuals who can offer encouragement, empathy, and practical assistance. Grant me the courage to

seek help and reach out when I need it. "Carry each other's burdens, and in this way, you will fulfill the law of Christ." - Galatians 6:2

5. Heavenly Father, I surrender any feelings of guilt or self-blame that may arise. Help me to recognize that post-partum depression is not my fault and that seeking help is a courageous act. Grant me the strength to seek professional assistance and support groups that can aid in my recovery. "Therefore confess your sins to each other and pray for each other so that you may be healed. The prayer of a righteous person is powerful and effective." - James 5:16

6. Lord, I pray for a renewed sense of purpose and joy in my role as a mother. Help me to see the beauty and significance of the everyday moments with my child. Fill my heart with gratitude and contentment, knowing that I am fulfilling a precious calling. "Children are a heritage from the Lord, offspring a reward from him." - Psalm 127:3

7. Gracious God, I surrender my worries and concerns about the future to You. Grant me peace in knowing that You are with me every step of the way. Help me to trust in Your plans and to find strength in Your promises. "For I know the plans I have for you," declares the Lord, "plans to prosper you and not to harm you, plans to give you hope and a future." - Jeremiah 29:11

SUNDAYS POST-PARTUM PRAYERS

1. Heavenly Father, I come before You with a heart full of gratitude. Thank You for bringing me safely through the journey of pregnancy and childbirth. I thank You for the gift of motherhood and the precious life You have entrusted to me. Help me to always be thankful and to see the blessings in every moment. "Give thanks to the Lord, for he is good; his love endures forever." - Psalm 107:1

2. Lord, I pray for an increase in faith during this post-partum period. Strengthen my trust in You and Your perfect plan for me and my child. Help me to rely on Your guidance and provision each day. "Trust in the Lord with all your heart and lean not on your own understanding." - Proverbs 3:5

3. Gracious God, I surrender my worries and anxieties to You. Help me to cast my burdens upon You, knowing that You care for me and my child. Grant me the peace that surpasses all understanding, guarding my heart and mind in Christ Jesus. "Do not be anxious about anything, but in every situation, by prayer and petition, with thanksgiving, present your requests to God." - Philippians 4:6

4. Lord, I pray for the wisdom and strength to be the best mother I can be. Guide me in making decisions that align with Your will and that benefit the well-being of my child. Help me to prioritize self-care and seek assistance when needed. "If any of you lacks wisdom, you should

ask God, who gives generously to all without finding fault, and it will be given to you." - James 1:5

5. Heavenly Father, I ask for Your divine help and intervention in all areas of my life. Help me to recognize when I need assistance and to reach out to others for support. Surround me with a community of believers who can uplift and encourage me on this journey. "Bear one another's burdens, and so fulfill the law of Christ." - Galatians 6:2

6. Lord, I pray for a deeper understanding of Your love and grace. Help me to extend grace to myself and to others, knowing that we are all imperfect beings in need of Your mercy. Fill my heart with compassion, kindness, and forgiveness. "Be kind and compassionate to one another, forgiving each other, just as in Christ God forgave you." - Ephesians 4:32

7. Gracious God, I surrender my desires, dreams, and plans to You. May Your will be done in my life and in the life of my child. Grant me the strength and courage to walk in obedience to Your Word, trusting that You have a purpose and a plan for us. "Commit your way to the Lord; trust in him, and he will act." - Psalm 37:5

CONCLUSION

As we come to the end of "Blessings in the Womb: A Prayer Handbook for Pregnant Women," I hope that this collection of prayers has been a source of comfort, guidance, and inspiration for expectant mothers. Pregnancy is a transformative and awe-inspiring time, and our hope is that this book has helped deepen your connection with God and provided a space for reflection, gratitude, and surrender.

Throughout the pages of this handbook, we have explored various aspects of pregnancy, addressing the physical, emotional, and spiritual dimensions. We have sought God's blessings, protection, and guidance for both mother and child, acknowledging the precious gift of life and the profound responsibility of nurturing it.

We have recognized the importance of prayer in fostering a closer walk with God during the pregnancy journey, relying on His strength, wisdom, and provision. We have offered prayers for good health, safe delivery, post-partum recovery, and the overall well-being of both mother and child.

It is my prayer that as you have engaged with these prayers, you have felt the presence of God in your life, bringing you peace, comfort, and assurance. We hope that you have found solace in His promises and experienced His faithfulness throughout every step of this miraculous journey.

As you continue your path through motherhood, remember that prayer is a powerful tool that can accompany you through every season of life. It is my hope that the habit of seeking God's presence through prayer will stay with you beyond the pregnancy period, becoming a lifelong source of strength, guidance, and peace.

May the words you have encountered in this prayer handbook continue to resonate in your heart, serving as a reminder of the incredible bond between a mother and her child, and the profound love and grace of our Heavenly Father. May these prayers be a source of inspiration and encouragement as you navigate the joys and challenges of motherhood.

I extend my heartfelt blessings to you, dear mothers, as you embark on this remarkable journey of motherhood. May God's grace continue to surround you and your child, may His wisdom guide your every step, and may His love sustain you through all the days of your life.

Another Olu Wonders wonderful book you might want to get is;

- Parents Pray for Yourself: An Everyday Handbook of Personal Prayer for Moms and Dads

- 365 Days of Blessings: A Parent's Prayer Handbook for Praying for Their Children

- The Wife and a Mother's Prayer Handbook

These are fantastic books you should get. You can also check out her other books for children, teenagers, and adults below.

ABOUT THE AUTHOR

Olu Wonders is an experienced minister in the prayer and children's ministry. She has authored numerous books catering to different age groups, reflecting her passion for nurturing the spiritual lives of children, teenagers, and adults. With a genuine love for God and a simple yet loving personality, Olu brings her deep understanding of prayer and ministry experience to inspire and guide readers on their spiritual journeys. Explore her books to deepen your understanding of God's love and grace and nourish your spirit.

We want to hear from you, send your testimonies and inquiries directly to contact: oluwonders123@gmail.com

BOOKS BY OLU WONDERS

For Children (Ages 0-12)

1. 365 Days of Bible Verses with Faith Confession for Children (Ages 0-12)

2. One-Year Journey of Weekly Bible Memory Verses for Children

3. Who Am I In Christ?

4. 365 Days Devotional for Children (Ages 0-12)

5. The Little Wisdom Book: Bible Proverbs for Children

6. Morning Prayers for Children

7. Afternoon Prayers for Children

8. Bedtime Prayers for Children

9. My ABC Book

10. My 123 Book

11. What Shall We Do Today? Christian Children Book

12. ABC Bible Character Book, Christian Children's Book

13. The Wonder Book: 4-in-1 Christian Children Story Book (Vol.1)

14. A-Z Animal Book for Children. (In English and Yoruba)

15. The Beatitude Book for Christian Children

16. The Fruits of the Holy Spirit; Christian Children's Book

17. Baby's and Toddler's First Prayer Book

18. The Lord is My Shephard, Christian Children's Book

19. Children Pray for Your Parents: Children Prayer Handbook for Praying for their Parents. (Ages 0-12)

20. Morning, Afternoon, and Bedtime for Children

For Teenagers (Ages 13-18)

21. Just for Young Ladies

22. The Burning Altar of Prayer Responsibility: The Price of Greatness

23. Responsibility: The Price of Greatness

24. 365 Days Teenagers Devotional (Ages 13-18)

25. Teenagers Pray for Your Parents: Teenagers Prayer Handbook for their Parents (Ages 13-18)

26. Morning, Afternoon, Bedtime, and Mid-Night Prayers for Teenagers

For Adults

27. Parents Pray for Yourself: An Everyday Handbook of Personal Prayer for Moms and Dads

28. 365 Days of Blessings: A Parent's Prayer Handbook for Praying for Their Children